# LECTIN-FREE

## DIET COOKBOOK

## FOR SENIORS

Delicious and Nourishing Recipes for Enhanced Health, Vitality, and Longevity

Kingsley Klopp

# Table of Contents

**Poultry Recipes**

# Important Note

Thank you for choosing the **Lectin-Free Diet Cookbook for Seniors**. We're delighted to have you join us on this journey towards better health and delicious, lectin-free dining. Before you dive into these wonderful recipes, we'd like to share a few important notes.

Every individual is unique, and dietary needs can vary widely from person to person. What works perfectly for one may not be ideal for another. That's why it's crucial to approach this cookbook as a flexible guide. Feel free to adjust the recipes to suit your personal health requirements and taste preferences. Your body knows best, so listen to it and make changes as needed.

If you ever find yourself uncertain about any dietary adjustments or if you have specific health concerns, we strongly encourage you to consult with your healthcare provider. Your doctor can offer personalized advice to ensure that any changes you make are safe and beneficial for you. This step is especially important if you're managing any chronic conditions or taking medications that could be affected by dietary changes.

Additionally, please note that the nutritional information provided with each recipe is approximate. The exact nutritional values can vary based on the specific ingredients you use and how you prepare your meals. Consider these figures as helpful guidelines rather than precise measurements.

Furthermore, If our cookbook has brought joy to your kitchen and table, we'd be thrilled to hear about your experiences in an Amazon review. On the flip side, if you stumble upon any hiccups while exploring our recipes, don't hesitate to get in touch at **kloppkingsley@gmail.com**. We're here to support your cooking journey every step of the way.

Our goal is to provide you with a collection of tasty, nutritious recipes that support your health and bring joy to your meals. We hope this cookbook becomes a valuable resource for you, helping you navigate the lectin-free lifestyle with ease and enjoyment.

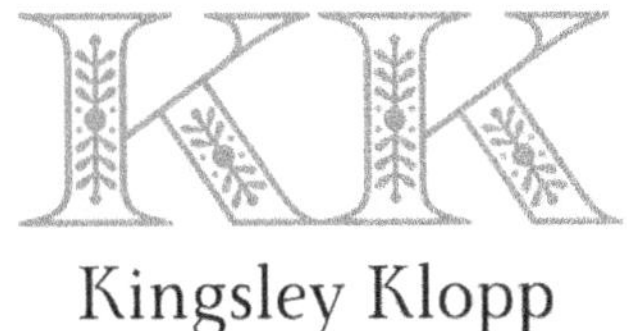

Kingsley Klopp

# Introduction

Welcome to the **Lectin-Free Diet Cookbook for Seniors**! If you've picked up this book, you're likely on a journey to improve your health, boost your energy, and enjoy life to the fullest—without the pesky interference of lectins. Whether you're new to the lectin-free lifestyle or looking for fresh, flavorful recipes to add to your collection, you're in the right place. We're about to set out on a culinary adventure that not only delights your taste buds but also supports your health and well-being.

Let's start by addressing the big question: *what exactly are lectins?* Lectins are a type of protein found in many plants, particularly in grains and legumes. While they can serve protective functions in plants, they can also cause digestive issues and inflammation in some people. For seniors, whose bodies might be more sensitive to these effects, reducing lectins in the diet can lead to improved digestion, reduced inflammation, and overall better health. But here's the great news: adopting a lectin-free diet doesn't mean you have to sacrifice flavor or enjoyment. Quite the opposite! This cookbook is packed with mouth-watering recipes that are both lectin-free and delicious. Imagine starting your day with a hearty breakfast that leaves you feeling energized and ready to tackle whatever comes your way. Picture yourself savoring a dinner that's not only satisfying but also gentle on your digestive system. We've designed this cookbook with seniors in mind. The recipes are straightforward, with easy-to-follow instructions and ingredients that are readily available. We understand that cooking should be a pleasure, not a chore, so we've kept things simple and fuss-free. Whether you're an experienced cook or a kitchen novice, you'll find these recipes accessible and enjoyable to make.

One of the key principles of this cookbook is the emphasis on whole, unprocessed foods. You'll discover a bounty of fruits, vegetables, lean proteins, and healthy fats that not only nourish your body but also help keep lectins at bay. Think vibrant salads bursting with fresh ingredients, comforting soups that warm your soul, and delectable desserts that you can indulge in without guilt. Food should be a source of joy and comfort, and we've infused that philosophy into every page of this cookbook. We also know that seniors have unique nutritional needs. As we age, maintaining a healthy diet becomes even more critical for preserving vitality and preventing chronic illnesses. This cookbook offers balanced meals that provide essential nutrients, promote heart health, support strong bones, and help manage weight. We've included tips on meal planning, shopping for the right ingredients, and making the most out of your meals.

But this book is more than just a collection of recipes. It's a guide to embracing a new way of eating that aligns with your body's needs. Each recipe comes with detailed instructions, nutritional information, and tips on how to make the most out of your meals. We've also included sections on understanding the benefits of a lectin-free diet, practical advice on shopping and meal prep, and strategies for making lasting changes to your eating habits.

So, let's get started! Grab your apron, head to the kitchen, and let's cook up some delicious, lectin-free meals together. Whether you're looking to alleviate digestive issues, reduce inflammation, or simply enjoy healthier meals, this cookbook is here to support you every step of the way. Let's turn the page on discomfort and embrace a new chapter of vibrant, flavorful, and healthy dining. Welcome to the **"Lectin-Free Diet Cookbook for Seniors"** – your new culinary adventure awaits!

# Chapter 1: Understanding Lectins

## *What Are Lectins?*

Lectins are a type of protein found in many plants and animal products. They play a crucial role in nature, acting as a defense mechanism for plants against pests and pathogens. However, when it comes to human consumption, lectins have garnered a lot of attention, often sparking debate among nutritionists and health enthusiasts. Understanding what lectins are, how they function, and their impact on our health is essential, especially for seniors looking to improve their well-being through diet.

### The Basics of Lectins

Lectins are a diverse group of proteins that can bind to carbohydrates. They are found in significant amounts in seeds, grains, legumes, and some vegetables. Common foods high in lectins include beans, lentils, peanuts, tomatoes, potatoes, and wheat. Lectins are often resistant to digestion and can pass through your gut unchanged. While this property helps plants deter pests, it can pose challenges to human digestion and health.

### The Dual Nature of Lectins

Lectins have a dual nature; they can be both beneficial and harmful. On the one hand, some lectins have medicinal properties. For example, certain lectins are being researched for their potential to fight cancer cells and improve immune function. On the other hand, high amounts of lectins can be toxic and may cause digestive issues or interfere with nutrient absorption.

For many, the harmful effects of lectins come into focus when discussing gut health. Lectins can bind to the gut lining, potentially causing inflammation and disrupting the balance of gut bacteria. This is particularly concerning for seniors, as the digestive system tends to become more sensitive with age. The symptoms can range from mild discomfort to more severe gastrointestinal issues, which can significantly affect the quality of life.

### Lectins and Autoimmune Responses

One of the most concerning aspects of lectins is their potential to trigger autoimmune responses. Autoimmune diseases occur when the body's immune system mistakenly attacks its own tissues. Lectins can bind to cell membranes and mimic the body's cells, confusing the immune system and leading it to attack its tissues. This can exacerbate conditions like rheumatoid arthritis, lupus, and other autoimmune disorders, which are already more prevalent among seniors.

**The Emotional Impact**

Imagine feeling constantly bloated, fatigued, or in pain, not knowing that the foods you eat might be contributing to your discomfort. For many seniors, dietary choices significantly impact their daily lives and overall well-being. Transitioning to a lectin-free diet can be a profound, emotional journey. It's about reclaiming control over one's health and finding relief from chronic ailments that may have plagued them for years. The joy of waking up without joint pain, the comfort of a settled stomach, and the energy to play with grandchildren are the rewards that await those who choose to explore a lectin-free lifestyle.

**Making Informed Choices**

Understanding lectins empowers individuals to make informed dietary choices. For some, reducing or eliminating high-lectin foods from their diet can lead to remarkable health improvements. Cooking methods can also reduce the lectin content in foods. Soaking, fermenting, sprouting, and pressure cooking are effective ways to diminish the lectin levels in beans, grains, and legumes, making them safer to consume.

**A Personal Reflection**

Reflect on the warmth of a family meal, the laughter around the dinner table, and the satisfaction of nourishing your body with food that truly benefits your health. As we age, the choices we make about our diet become increasingly significant. Adopting a lectin-free diet isn't just about avoiding certain foods; it's about embracing a lifestyle that prioritizes health and well-being. It's about finding joy in meals that heal, rather than harm. It's about living each day with the vitality and happiness that every senior deserves.

In summary, lectins are a fascinating yet complex component of our diet. While they play a natural role in plant defense, their impact on human health is significant and multifaceted. For seniors, particularly, understanding and managing lectin intake can lead to a dramatic improvement in health and quality of life. Embracing a lectin-free diet is not just a nutritional choice; it's a step towards a healthier, happier future. By making informed decisions and listening to our bodies, we can find a balance that allows us to enjoy food without compromising our well-being.

# *Health Effects of Lectins*

**The Beneficial Effects of Lectins**

Lectins are not inherently harmful; in fact, some lectins have significant health benefits. They have been studied for their potential anti-cancer properties. Certain lectins can recognize and bind to cancer cells, potentially inhibiting their growth or promoting their destruction. This property is being explored in medical research to develop new cancer therapies.

Moreover, some lectins have been found to possess antimicrobial properties, helping to protect against bacterial infections. They can enhance the immune response, contributing to the body's ability to fight off pathogens. Additionally, lectins in foods like legumes and whole grains are associated with various health benefits, including reduced risks of cardiovascular diseases and improved glycemic control. These benefits are primarily due to the high fiber content and nutrient density of these foods, which contribute to overall health and well-being.

**The Harmful Effects of Lectins**

Despite their potential benefits, lectins can also have adverse effects on health, particularly when consumed in large quantities or when not properly prepared. Here are some of the key health concerns associated with lectins:

1. **Digestive Issues:** Lectins are known to interfere with digestion. They can resist breakdown by digestive enzymes and pass through the gastrointestinal tract unchanged. In the gut, they can bind to the lining of the intestine, potentially causing irritation and inflammation. This can lead to symptoms such as bloating, gas, diarrhea, and abdominal pain. For individuals with sensitive digestive systems, such as seniors, these effects can be particularly troublesome.

2. **Nutrient Absorption:** Lectins can bind to nutrients and interfere with their absorption in the gut. This is particularly concerning for essential minerals like calcium, iron, zinc, and magnesium. Over time, this can lead to nutrient deficiencies, which can have various health implications, including weakened immunity, anemia, and impaired bone health. Seniors, who already face challenges in maintaining optimal nutrient levels, may be at higher risk.

3. **Leaky Gut Syndrome:** Chronic consumption of high-lectin foods has been linked to increased intestinal permeability, also known as "leaky gut" syndrome. This condition occurs when the tight junctions between intestinal cells become loose, allowing undigested food particles, toxins, and microbes to enter the bloodstream. This can trigger systemic inflammation and contribute to the development of autoimmune diseases, where the immune system mistakenly attacks the body's tissues.

**4. Autoimmune Reactions:** Lectins can mimic proteins in the body, potentially confusing the immune system. This molecular mimicry can lead to autoimmune responses, where the body starts attacking its tissues. Conditions such as rheumatoid arthritis, lupus, and multiple sclerosis have been linked to dietary lectins. For seniors, who are more susceptible to autoimmune diseases, managing lectin intake can be crucial in controlling symptoms and improving quality of life.

**5. Allergic Reactions:** Some individuals may be allergic to specific lectins. These allergic reactions can range from mild symptoms like itching and rashes to severe anaphylactic responses. Identifying and avoiding foods that trigger allergic reactions is essential for those with known sensitivities.

## Mitigating the Harmful Effects of Lectins

To enjoy the benefits of lectin-rich foods while minimizing their harmful effects, it is important to prepare them properly. Cooking methods such as soaking, fermenting, sprouting, and pressure cooking can significantly reduce the lectin content in foods. For example, soaking beans overnight and cooking them thoroughly can deactivate most of the harmful lectins, making them safe to consume. Incorporating a variety of lectin-free or low-lectin foods into the diet can also help balance nutrient intake and reduce potential negative impacts. Foods such as leafy greens, cruciferous vegetables, pasture-raised meats, and certain fruits are nutritious options that are low in lectins.

Hence, lectins are a double-edged sword in the world of nutrition. While they offer potential health benefits, their adverse effects cannot be ignored, especially for seniors who may be more vulnerable to digestive and autoimmune issues.

# Common Foods High in Lectins

Lectins are naturally occurring proteins found in a wide variety of foods, primarily plants. These proteins can bind to carbohydrates and play a role in plant defense mechanisms against pests and pathogens. While lectins can offer some health benefits, they can also cause digestive issues and other health problems, particularly when consumed in large quantities or not properly prepared. For seniors and those with sensitive digestive systems, being aware of foods high in lectins is important for managing health and well-being. Let us look at some of the most common lectin-rich foods and their impact on health.

**Legumes**

Legumes are among the most well-known sources of lectins. This category includes beans, lentils, chickpeas, and peanuts. They are nutrient-dense and provide significant health benefits, such as high fiber, protein, and essential vitamins and minerals. However, they also contain high levels of lectins, which can pose digestive challenges.

- Beans: Kidney beans, black beans, and soybeans are particularly high in lectins. Raw or undercooked beans can cause severe digestive distress, including nausea, vomiting, and diarrhea, due to the presence of a lectin called phytohemagglutinin. Proper cooking, such as soaking beans overnight and then boiling them for at least 10 minutes, can significantly reduce lectin content.
- Lentils: While lentils are easier to digest than some other legumes, they still contain lectins. Soaking and thoroughly cooking lentils can reduce their lectin levels and make them safer to eat.
- Peanuts: Peanuts are not only a common allergen but also contain lectins that can affect digestion and nutrient absorption. Roasting peanuts can reduce lectin levels, but those with sensitive digestive systems should consume them in moderation.

**Grains**

Grains are another major source of lectins, particularly those in the seeds and outer bran layers. Modern diets are often rich in grains, which can contribute to lectin intake.

- Wheat: Wheat contains wheat germ agglutinin (WGA), a lectin that can cause digestive issues and interfere with nutrient absorption. WGA is resistant to heat and digestive enzymes, making it a concern even in cooked wheat products like bread and pasta.
- Rice: Brown rice, which retains its bran layer, contains more lectins than white rice. Soaking and cooking rice can help reduce lectin content, but some individuals may still experience sensitivity.
- Barley and Rye: These grains also contain significant amounts of lectins. Fermentation, as used in sourdough bread, can help reduce lectin levels and make these grains more digestible.

**Vegetables**

Certain vegetables, especially those in the nightshade family, are high in lectins. These vegetables are nutritious but can cause problems for some individuals.

- Tomatoes: Tomatoes contain lectins primarily in their skins and seeds. Cooking tomatoes can reduce lectin content, making them easier to digest for those with sensitivities.
- Potatoes: Potatoes, particularly their skins, contain lectins. Cooking potatoes thoroughly can reduce lectin levels, but individuals with lectin sensitivities should consider peeling them before consumption.
- Eggplants: Another member of the nightshade family, eggplants contain lectins that can cause digestive issues. Cooking and removing the skins can help mitigate these effects.

**Dairy**

Some dairy products contain lectins, particularly those derived from animals fed a diet high in lectin-containing grains.

- Milk: Conventional milk can contain lectins if the cows were fed grain-based diets. Switching to milk from grass-fed cows or opting for fermented dairy products like yogurt and kefir can reduce lectin intake.
- Cheese: Hard cheeses, particularly those made from grain-fed animals, can contain lectins. Fermented cheeses may have lower lectin levels due to the fermentation process.

**Nuts and Seeds**

Nuts and seeds are nutrient-dense foods that also contain lectins. While they offer numerous health benefits, they can be problematic for those sensitive to lectins.

- Almonds: Raw almonds contain lectins, particularly in their skins. Soaking and roasting almonds can reduce lectin levels.
- Sunflower Seeds: These seeds are a common snack but also contain lectins. Opting for soaked or sprouted sunflower seeds can help reduce lectin content.

**Fruits**

Certain fruits contain lectins, although they are generally lower in lectin content compared to other food groups.

- Bananas: Bananas contain lectins, particularly in their peels. However, the edible part of the fruit has lower levels, making it generally safe for most people.
- Melons: Watermelons and cantaloupes have lectins, especially in their seeds and rinds. The flesh of these fruits is lower in lectins and usually safe to consume.

**Managing Lectin Intake**

To minimize the potential negative effects of lectins, proper food preparation is key. Methods such as soaking, sprouting, fermenting, and cooking can significantly reduce the lectin content in many foods. For those particularly sensitive to lectins, avoiding high-lectin foods or opting for low-lectin alternatives can be beneficial.

# *Steps to Eliminate Lectins from Your Diet*

**Understanding the Role of Lectins**

Lectins are proteins found in many plants, particularly in seeds, grains, legumes, and some vegetables. While they serve as a defense mechanism for plants, lectins can be hard on the human digestive system, causing inflammation and interfering with nutrient absorption. For many people, especially seniors, reducing or eliminating lectins from the diet can lead to significant health improvements.

**Step 1: Identify High-Lectin Foods**

The first step in eliminating lectins from your diet is to identify the foods that are high in these proteins. Common high-lectin foods include:

- Legumes: Beans (kidney, black, soy), lentils, chickpeas, peanuts
- Grains: Wheat, barley, rye, quinoa, brown rice
- Nightshade Vegetables: Tomatoes, potatoes, eggplants, bell peppers
- Dairy: Products from grain-fed animals
- Fruits: Bananas, melons
- Nuts and Seeds: Almonds, sunflower seeds

Understanding which foods contain high levels of lectins will help you make more informed dietary choices.

**Step 2: Transition Gradually**

Transitioning to a lectin-free diet should be done gradually to allow your body to adjust. Sudden changes can cause digestive distress or nutrient imbalances. Start by eliminating one category of high-lectin foods at a time. For example, you could begin by cutting out legumes, then grains, followed by nightshade vegetables, and so on.

**Step 3: Focus on Low-Lectin Foods**

While eliminating high-lectin foods, it's essential to incorporate low-lectin alternatives to maintain a balanced and nutritious diet. Some low-lectin foods include:

- Vegetables: Leafy greens (spinach, kale), cruciferous vegetables (broccoli, cauliflower), onions, garlic
- Fruits: Berries (blueberries, strawberries), apples, citrus fruits
- Animal Products: Grass-fed meats, pasture-raised poultry, wild-caught fish
- Dairy Alternatives: Milk from grass-fed animals, coconut milk, almond milk (soaked almonds)
- Healthy Fats: Olive oil, coconut oil, avocado oil

These foods are nutrient-dense and can help you maintain a healthy diet while avoiding lectins.

**Step 4: Proper Preparation Methods**

If you want to enjoy some high-lectin foods occasionally, proper preparation methods can help reduce their lectin content:

- Soaking: Soak beans, grains, and nuts overnight. This helps to reduce the lectin content and makes them easier to digest.
- Sprouting: Sprouting grains, legumes, and seeds can significantly lower their lectin levels.
- Fermenting: Fermentation breaks down lectins and other anti-nutrients, making foods like sourdough bread and fermented vegetables safer to eat.
- Pressure Cooking: Pressure cooking is highly effective at reducing lectins in beans, legumes, and certain vegetables. Ensure you follow recommended cooking times to maximize the reduction of lectins.

**Step 5: Monitor Your Health**

As you eliminate lectins from your diet, monitor your health closely. Keep a food diary to track what you eat and note any changes in your symptoms. Pay attention to improvements in digestive health, energy levels, and overall well-being. This can help you identify which foods you may need to avoid permanently and which ones you can occasionally reintroduce.

**Step 6: Supplement Wisely**

While transitioning to a lectin-free diet, ensure you are getting all the essential nutrients. Some high-lectin foods are rich in vitamins and minerals, so you may need to find alternative sources or consider supplements. For example:

- Calcium: If you reduce dairy, consider alternative sources like leafy greens, fortified plant milks, or a calcium supplement.
- Iron and Zinc: If you cut back on beans and grains, include more red meat, poultry, seafood, and nuts (like soaked almonds) in your diet.
- Fiber: Ensure you get enough fiber from low-lectin vegetables, fruits, and seeds like chia and flax.

**Step 7: Seek Professional Guidance**

Consulting with a healthcare professional, such as a dietitian or nutritionist, can provide personalized guidance and support. They can help you create a balanced meal plan, ensure you are meeting your nutritional needs, and offer strategies to manage any health conditions effectively.

**Step 8: Stay Informed and Flexible**

The science of nutrition is always evolving, and new information about lectins and their effects on health continues to emerge. Stay informed by reading up-to-date research and expert opinions. Be flexible and willing to adjust your diet as needed based on new information and your personal health experiences.

# Shopping Guide for Lectin-Free Foods

**Understanding Lectin-Free Foods**

Lectin-free foods are those that either contain no lectins or have minimal lectin content that can be further reduced through proper preparation methods. These foods can be broadly categorized into vegetables, fruits, proteins, dairy alternatives, grains and legumes substitutes, nuts and seeds, and healthy fats.

**Vegetables**

When shopping for vegetables, focus on those that are low in lectins and rich in nutrients. Here are some excellent choices:

- Leafy Greens: Spinach, kale, Swiss chard, and lettuce are all low in lectins and packed with vitamins and minerals.
- Cruciferous Vegetables: Broccoli, cauliflower, Brussels sprouts, and cabbage are nutritious and low in lectins.
- Alliums: Garlic, onions, leeks, and shallots add flavor to your meals without the lectin content.
- Other Low-Lectin Veggies: Asparagus, cucumbers, celery, mushrooms, and zucchini are all safe and healthy options.

**Shopping Tips:**

- Choose fresh, organic vegetables when possible to avoid pesticides and other chemicals.
- Frozen vegetables can be a good alternative when fresh produce is not available. Ensure they are plain and not mixed with high-lectin ingredients.

**Fruits**

Fruits can be a delightful part of a lectin-free diet, especially those lower in lectins:

- Berries: Blueberries, strawberries, raspberries, and blackberries are all low in lectins and high in antioxidants.
- Citrus Fruits: Oranges, lemons, limes, and grapefruits are excellent choices.
- Other Low-Lectin Fruits: Apples, pears, peaches, and cherries are generally safe to consume.

**Shopping Tips:**

- Opt for fresh, organic fruits to reduce exposure to pesticides.
- Choose whole fruits over dried or processed versions to avoid added sugars and preservatives.

**Proteins**

Proteins are essential for a balanced diet. Focus on high-quality, low-lectin protein sources:

- Meat and Poultry: Grass-fed beef, pasture-raised chicken, and turkey are ideal. These animals are typically fed diets low in lectins.
- Seafood: Wild-caught fish such as salmon, cod, and sardines are excellent protein sources.
- Eggs: Pasture-raised eggs are low in lectins and provide essential nutrients.

**Shopping Tips:**

- Look for labels such as "grass-fed," "pasture-raised," and "wild-caught" to ensure the highest quality.
- Buy fresh, unprocessed meats and seafood to avoid additives and preservatives.

**Dairy Alternatives**

While dairy can contain lectins if the animals are grain-fed, there are many lectin-free alternatives:

- Milk: Opt for coconut milk or almond milk (ensure the almonds have been soaked and peeled).
- Cheese: Cheese made from the milk of grass-fed animals or dairy-free options like nut-based cheeses.
- Yogurt: Coconut yogurt or almond milk yogurt are good alternatives.

**Shopping Tips:**

- Read labels carefully to avoid additives and preservatives.
- Choose unsweetened versions to avoid added sugars.

**Grains and Legume Substitutes**

Traditional grains and legumes are high in lectins, but there are excellent substitutes available:

- Grain Substitutes: Cauliflower rice, cassava flour, coconut flour, and almond flour are great alternatives.
- Legume Substitutes: Green beans and peas are lower in lectins and can be enjoyed in moderation.

**Shopping Tips:**

- Look for gluten-free labels to avoid wheat-based products.
- Experiment with different flour substitutes for baking and cooking.

**Nuts and Seeds**

Nuts and seeds can be part of a lectin-free diet when properly prepared:

- Low-Lectin Nuts: Macadamia nuts, pecans, and walnuts are good choices.
- Seeds: Chia seeds and flaxseeds are low in lectins and offer valuable nutrients.

**Shopping Tips:**

- Buy raw nuts and seeds and soak or sprout them before consumption.
- Avoid nuts and seeds that have been roasted in unhealthy oils.

**Healthy Fats**

Healthy fats are crucial for a balanced diet and can enhance the absorption of fat-soluble vitamins:

- Oils: Extra virgin olive oil, avocado oil, and coconut oil are all low in lectins and healthy.
- Avocados: A great source of healthy fats and low in lectins.

**Shopping Tips:**

- Choose oils that are cold-pressed and unrefined for the best quality.
- Store oils in a cool, dark place to prevent them from going rancid.

**General Shopping Tips**

1. Plan Your Meals: Before heading to the store, plan your meals for the week. This will help you create a focused shopping list and avoid impulse buys.
2. Read Labels Carefully: Many processed foods contain hidden lectins or other unwanted ingredients. Reading labels ensures you know exactly what you're buying.
3. Shop the Perimeter: The perimeter of the grocery store typically has fresh produce, meats, and dairy, while the inner aisles often contain processed foods.
4. Buy in Bulk: For items like nuts, seeds, and grains substitutes, buying in bulk can save money and ensure you always have lectin-free options on hand.
5. Seasonal and Local Produce: Choosing seasonal and local produce can enhance nutrient intake and reduce the environmental impact.

# Further Clarification

We'd like to reiterate an important point: while the recipes in this book are designed to be lectin-free, you may encounter some ingredients that naturally contain lectins. Please do not be alarmed or confused. The reason for this inclusion is simple—everyone's dietary needs are unique, and what works wonders for one person might not be the best fit for another. We believe in providing a flexible approach that allows you to tailor the recipes to your individual health requirements and preferences.

Furthermore, the cooking methods we have employed are specifically designed to minimize the lectin content in these ingredients as much as possible. Techniques such as soaking, fermenting, and pressure cooking are used to reduce lectins to the lowest feasible levels, ensuring that you can enjoy these dishes with confidence and comfort.

Our goal is to offer you a variety of delicious, nutritious recipes that support your health and enhance your culinary experience. We encourage you to adapt these recipes to meet your personal needs and consult with your healthcare provider if you have any questions or concerns.

# Breakfast Recipes

**Watercress Soup**

**Ingredients:**

- 2 tablespoons extra virgin olive oil
- 1 large onion, chopped
- 2 cloves garlic, minced
- 4 cups watercress, washed and chopped
- 4 cups low-sodium vegetable broth
- 1 medium sweet potato, peeled and diced
- 1 teaspoon sea salt
- 1/2 teaspoon ground white pepper
- 1/4 cup fresh parsley, chopped

**Instructions:**

1. In a large pot, heat the olive oil over medium heat.
2. Add the chopped onion and garlic, sautéing until the onion becomes translucent, about 5 minutes.
3. Add the sweet potato and cook for another 5 minutes, stirring occasionally.
4. Pour in the vegetable broth and bring to a boil. Reduce heat and simmer until the sweet potato is tender, about 15 minutes.
5. Add the watercress to the pot and cook for another 5 minutes.
6. Using an immersion blender, puree the soup until smooth. Alternatively, transfer the soup to a blender in batches and blend until smooth.
7. Season with sea salt and ground white pepper.
8. Serve hot, garnished with fresh parsley.

**Nutrition Info (Per Serving):**

- Calories: 110
- Protein: 2g
- Carbohydrates: 17g
- Fat: 4g
- Fiber: **3g**

**Serves: 4**

**Cooking Time: 30 minutes**

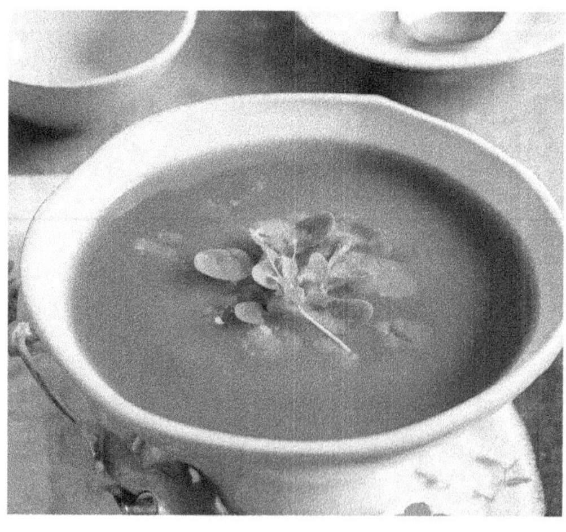

**Herb Roasted Chicken Thighs**

**Ingredients:**

- 4 bone-in, skin-on chicken thighs
- 2 tablespoons extra virgin olive oil
- 1 tablespoon fresh rosemary, chopped
- 1 tablespoon fresh thyme, chopped
- 1 tablespoon fresh oregano, chopped
- 1 teaspoon sea salt
- 1/2 teaspoon ground black pepper
- 2 cloves garlic, minced
- Juice of 1 lemon

**Instructions:**

1. Preheat the oven to 400°F (200°C).
2. In a small bowl, combine the olive oil, rosemary, thyme, oregano, sea salt, black pepper, garlic, and lemon juice.
3. Rub the mixture evenly over the chicken thighs.
4. Place the chicken thighs on a baking sheet lined with parchment paper.
5. Roast in the preheated oven for 35-40 minutes, or until the chicken reaches an internal temperature of 165°F (74°C) and the skin is crispy.
6. Remove from the oven and let rest for 5 minutes before serving.

**Nutrition Info (Per Serving):**

- Calories: 280
- Protein: 25g
- Carbohydrates: 1g
- Fat: 20g
- Fiber: **0g**

**Serves: 4**
**Cooking Time: 45 minutes**

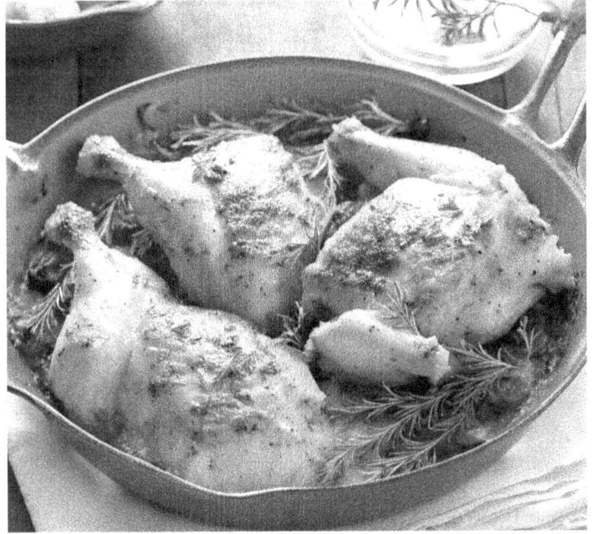

**Radish and Smoked Salmon Plate**

**Ingredients:**

- 4 radishes, thinly sliced
- 4 ounces smoked salmon
- 1 avocado, sliced
- 2 tablespoons capers, drained
- 1 tablespoon extra virgin olive oil
- 1 teaspoon fresh dill, chopped
- 1 teaspoon lemon zest
- 1/2 teaspoon sea salt
- 1/4 teaspoon ground black pepper

**Instructions:**

1. Arrange the radish slices on a serving plate.
2. Layer the smoked salmon and avocado slices on top of the radishes.
3. Sprinkle the capers over the plate.
4. Drizzle with olive oil and sprinkle with fresh dill and lemon zest.
5. Season with sea salt and ground black pepper.
6. Serve immediately.

**Nutrition Info (Per Serving):**

- Calories: 210
- Protein: 12g
- Carbohydrates: 6g
- Fat: 16g
- Fiber: 4g

**Serves: 2**
**Cooking Time: 10 minutes**

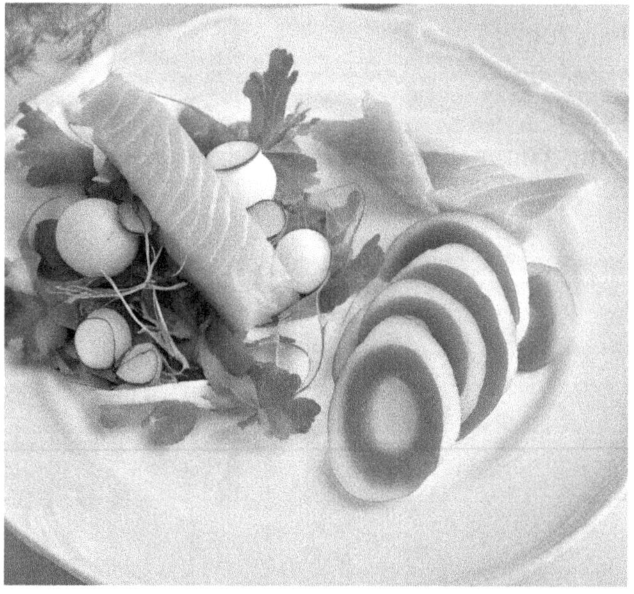

**Hard-Boiled Eggs with Olive Oil Drizzle**

**Ingredients:**

- 4 large eggs
- 2 tablespoons extra virgin olive oil
- 1 teaspoon sea salt
- 1/2 teaspoon smoked paprika
- 1 teaspoon fresh parsley, chopped

**Instructions:**

1. Place the eggs in a saucepan and cover with cold water.
2. Bring the water to a boil over medium-high heat. Once boiling, reduce heat to low and let simmer for 10 minutes.
3. Remove the eggs from the hot water and transfer them to a bowl of ice water to cool for 5 minutes.
4. Peel the eggs and slice them in half.
5. Arrange the egg halves on a serving plate.
6. Drizzle with olive oil and sprinkle with sea salt and smoked paprika.
7. Garnish with fresh parsley and serve.

**Nutrition Info (Per Serving):**

- Calories: 160
- Protein: 12g
- Carbohydrates: 1g
- Fat: 12g
- Fiber: 0g

**Serves: 2**
**Cooking Time: 15 minutes**

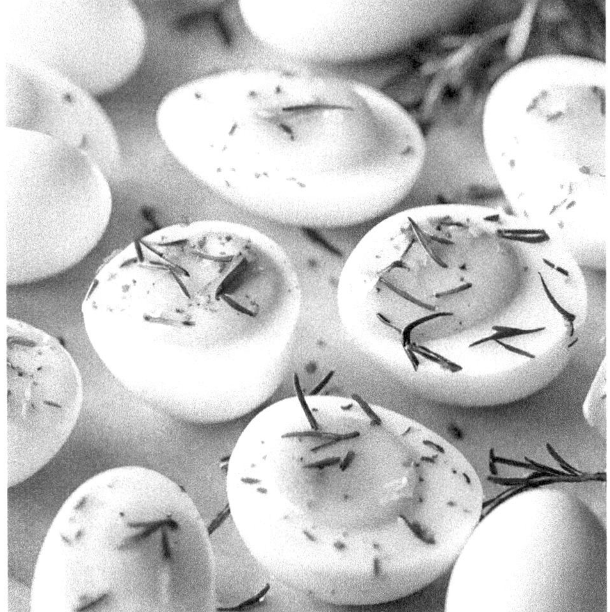

## 5. Tuna and Olive Salad

**Ingredients:**

- 1 can (5 ounces) tuna in olive oil, drained
- 1/4 cup green olives, sliced
- 1/4 cup black olives, sliced
- 1/4 cup red onion, finely chopped
- 1 avocado, diced
- 2 tablespoons extra virgin olive oil
- 1 tablespoon lemon juice
- 1 teaspoon Dijon mustard
- 1 teaspoon fresh parsley, chopped
- 1/2 teaspoon sea salt
- 1/4 teaspoon ground black pepper

**Instructions:**

1. In a large bowl, combine the tuna, green olives, black olives, red onion, and avocado.
2. In a small bowl, whisk together the olive oil, lemon juice, Dijon mustard, parsley, sea salt, and black pepper.
3. Pour the dressing over the tuna mixture and toss gently to combine.
4. Serve immediately or chill for 30 minutes to let the flavors meld.

**Nutrition Info (Per Serving):**

- Calories: 300
- Protein: 18g
- Carbohydrates: 8g
- Fat: 23g
- Fiber: 5g

**Serves: 2**

**Cooking Time: 10** minutes

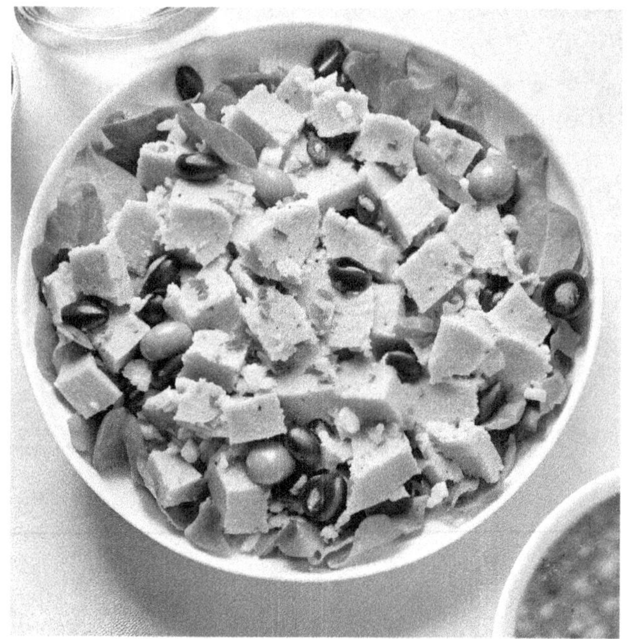

**6. Macadamia Nut Butter on Celery**

**Ingredients:**

- 1/2 cup macadamia nuts
- 4 large celery stalks, cut into 3-inch pieces
- 1 tablespoon extra virgin olive oil
- 1 teaspoon honey (optional)
- 1/4 teaspoon sea salt

**Instructions:**

1. In a food processor, blend the macadamia nuts and olive oil until smooth. Add honey if desired and continue blending until well combined.
2. Spread the macadamia nut butter on the celery pieces.
3. Sprinkle with sea salt and serve.

**Nutrition Info (Per Serving):**

- Calories: 250
- Protein: 3g
- Carbohydrates: 6g
- Fat: 24g
- Fiber: 3g

**Serves: 2**

**Cooking Time: 10** minutes

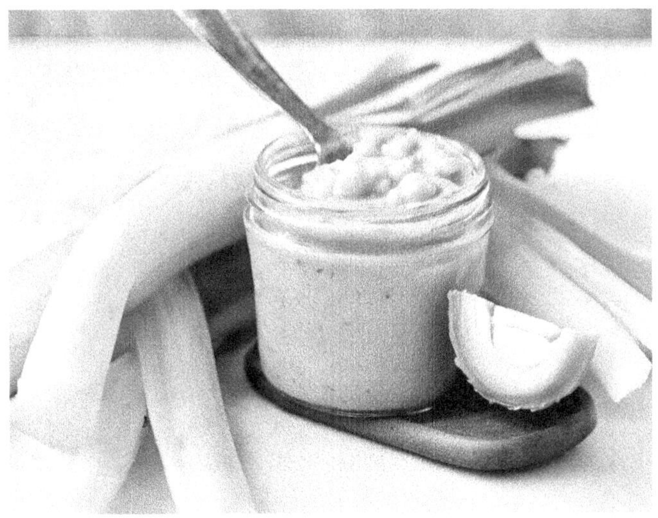

# 7. Olive Tapenade with Endive Leaves

## Ingredients:

- 1 cup mixed olives (green and black), pitted
- 2 cloves garlic, minced
- 2 tablespoons capers, drained
- 1 tablespoon fresh lemon juice
- 1 tablespoon fresh parsley, chopped
- 2 tablespoons extra virgin olive oil
- 1/2 teaspoon sea salt
- 1/4 teaspoon ground black pepper
- 2 heads of endive, leaves separated

## Instructions:

1. In a food processor, combine the olives, garlic, capers, lemon juice, parsley, olive oil, sea salt, and black pepper.
2. Pulse until the mixture is coarsely chopped and well combined.
3. Spoon the tapenade onto the endive leaves.
4. Arrange on a platter and serve.

## Nutrition Info (Per Serving):

- Calories: 180
- Protein: 2g
- Carbohydrates: 5g
- Fat: 17g
- Fiber: 2g

**Serves: 4**
**Cooking Time: 10 minutes**

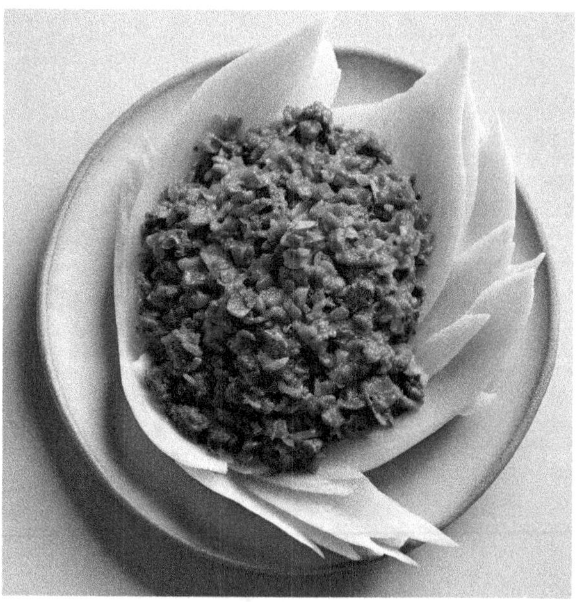

## 8. Sliced Turkey and Cucumber

**Ingredients:**

- 8 slices of roasted turkey breast
- 1 large cucumber, thinly sliced
- 2 tablespoons extra virgin olive oil
- 1 tablespoon apple cider vinegar
- 1 teaspoon fresh dill, chopped
- 1/2 teaspoon sea salt
- 1/4 teaspoon ground black pepper

**Instructions:**

1. Arrange the turkey slices and cucumber slices on a serving platter.
2. In a small bowl, whisk together the olive oil, apple cider vinegar, dill, sea salt, and black pepper.
3. Drizzle the dressing over the turkey and cucumber.
4. Serve immediately.

**Nutrition Info (Per Serving):**

- Calories: 150
- Protein: 15g
- Carbohydrates: 4g
- Fat: 8g
- Fiber: 1g

**Serves: 2**
**Cooking Time: 5 minutes**

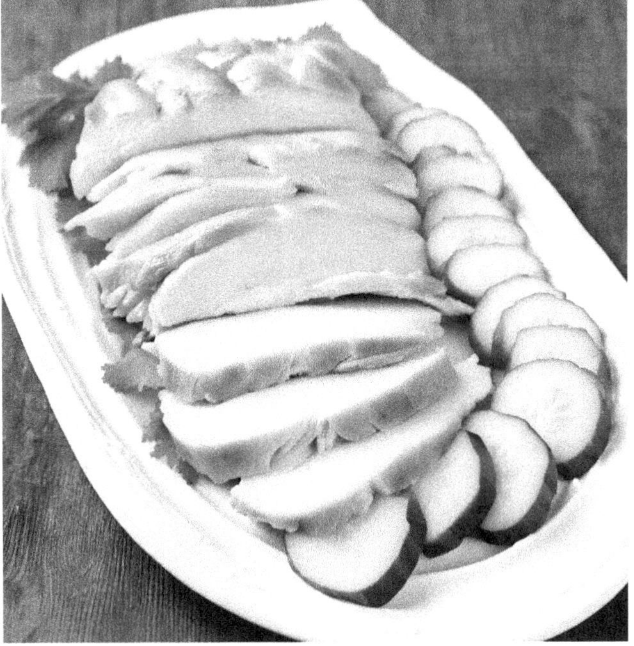

## 9. Lemon and Herb Chicken Drumsticks

**Ingredients:**

- 8 chicken drumsticks
- 1/4 cup extra virgin olive oil
- Juice of 2 lemons
- 2 cloves garlic, minced
- 1 tablespoon fresh rosemary, chopped
- 1 tablespoon fresh thyme, chopped
- 1 teaspoon sea salt
- 1/2 teaspoon ground black pepper

**Instructions:**

1. Preheat the oven to 400°F (200°C).
2. In a large bowl, whisk together the olive oil, lemon juice, garlic, rosemary, thyme, sea salt, and black pepper.
3. Add the chicken drumsticks to the bowl and toss to coat.
4. Arrange the drumsticks on a baking sheet lined with parchment paper.
5. Bake for 35-40 minutes, or until the chicken reaches an internal temperature of 165°F (74°C).
6. Remove from the oven and let rest for 5 minutes before serving.

**Nutrition Info (Per Serving):**

- Calories: 250
- Protein: 20g
- Carbohydrates: 2g
- Fat: 18g
- Fiber: 1g

**Serves: 4**

**Cooking Time: 45 minutes**

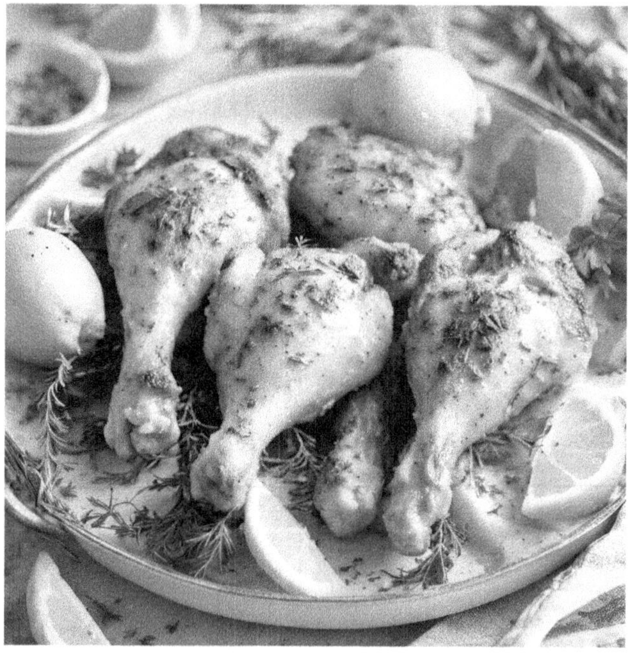

## 10. Pistachio and Pumpkin Seed Granola

**Ingredients:**

- 1 cup pistachios, shelled and chopped
- 1 cup pumpkin seeds
- 1/2 cup coconut flakes
- 1/4 cup chia seeds
- 1/4 cup flaxseeds
- 2 tablespoons extra virgin olive oil
- 1/4 cup honey or maple syrup
- 1 teaspoon vanilla extract
- 1/2 teaspoon sea salt
- 1/2 teaspoon ground cinnamon

**Instructions:**

1. Preheat the oven to 300°F (150°C).
2. In a large bowl, combine the pistachios, pumpkin seeds, coconut flakes, chia seeds, and flaxseeds.
3. In a small saucepan, heat the olive oil, honey (or maple syrup), and vanilla extract over low heat until well combined.
4. Pour the wet mixture over the dry ingredients and stir to coat.
5. Spread the granola mixture evenly on a baking sheet lined with parchment paper.
6. Sprinkle with sea salt and ground cinnamon.
7. Bake for 20-25 minutes, stirring halfway through, until golden brown.
8. Allow the granola to cool completely before storing in an airtight container.

**Nutrition Info (Per Serving):**

- Calories: 220
- Protein: 6g
- Carbohydrates: 15g
- Fat: 16g
- Fiber: 4g

**Serves: 8**
**Cooking Time: 30** minutes

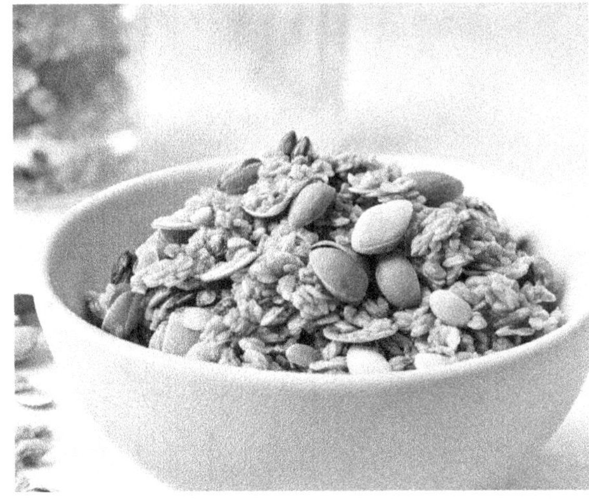

## 11. Mustard Greens and Bacon Stir-Fry

**Ingredients:**

- 6 slices bacon, chopped
- 1 large bunch mustard greens, washed and chopped
- 1 onion, thinly sliced
- 2 cloves garlic, minced
- 1 tablespoon apple cider vinegar
- 1/2 teaspoon sea salt
- 1/4 teaspoon ground black pepper

**Instructions:**

1. In a large skillet, cook the bacon over medium heat until crispy. Remove the bacon with a slotted spoon and set aside, leaving the bacon fat in the skillet.
2. Add the onion to the skillet and sauté until translucent, about 5 minutes.
3. Add the garlic and cook for another 1 minute.
4. Add the mustard greens to the skillet and cook until wilted, about 5-7 minutes.
5. Stir in the apple cider vinegar, sea salt, and black pepper.
6. Return the cooked bacon to the skillet and stir to combine.
7. Serve hot.

**Nutrition Info (Per Serving):**

- Calories: 150
- Protein: 6g
- Carbohydrates: 6g
- Fat: 12g
- Fiber: 3g

**Serves: 4**

**Cooking Time: 20 minutes**

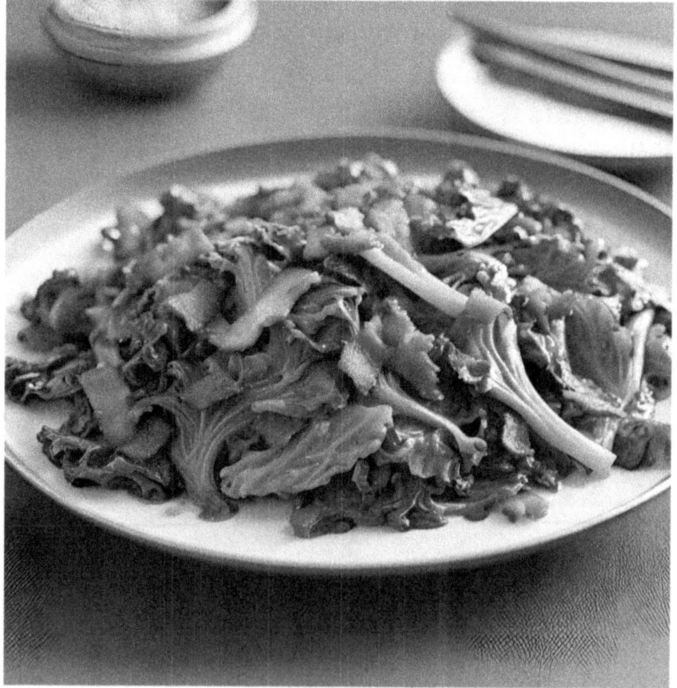

**12. Herbal Tea with Coconut Oil**

**Ingredients:**

- 2 cups water
- 1 herbal tea bag (chamomile, peppermint, or your choice)
- 1 tablespoon coconut oil
- 1 teaspoon honey (optional)
- 1 slice lemon (optional)

**Instructions:**

1. Bring the water to a boil in a small saucepan.
2. Remove from heat and steep the herbal tea bag in the hot water for 5-7 minutes.
3. Remove the tea bag and stir in the coconut oil until melted.
4. Add honey and lemon slice if desired.
5. Pour into a mug and serve hot.

**Nutrition Info (Per Serving):**

- Calories: 100
- Protein: 0g
- Carbohydrates: 1g
- Fat: 11g
- Fiber: 0g

**Serves: 2**
**Cooking Time: 10 minutes**

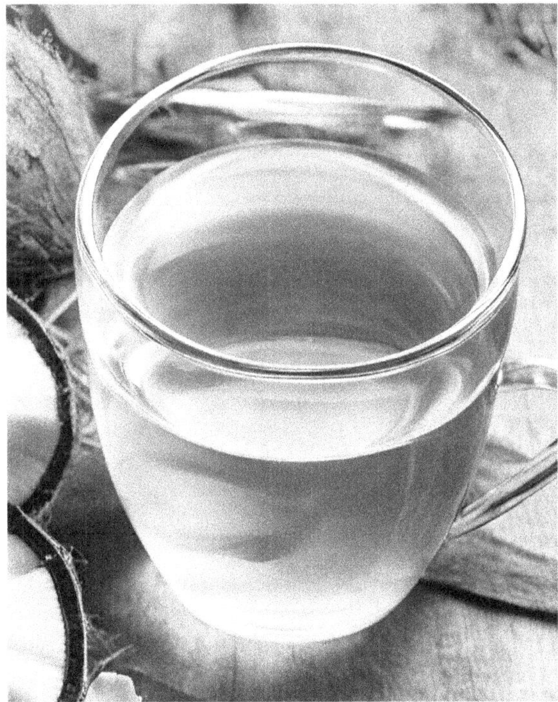

## 13. Cinnamon Coconut Latte

**Ingredients:**

- 1 cup coconut milk
- 1/2 cup brewed coffee
- 1 tablespoon coconut oil
- 1 teaspoon ground cinnamon
- 1 teaspoon vanilla extract
- 1 teaspoon honey (optional)

**Instructions:**

1. In a small saucepan, heat the coconut milk over medium heat until warm.
2. Add the brewed coffee, coconut oil, cinnamon, and vanilla extract to the saucepan.
3. Stir until the coconut oil is melted and the mixture is well combined.
4. Pour into a mug and sweeten with honey if desired.
5. Serve hot.

**Nutrition Info (Per Serving):**

- Calories: 180
- Protein: 1g
- Carbohydrates: 4g
- Fat: 18g
- Fiber: 1g

**Serves: 1**

**Cooking Time: 10 minutes**

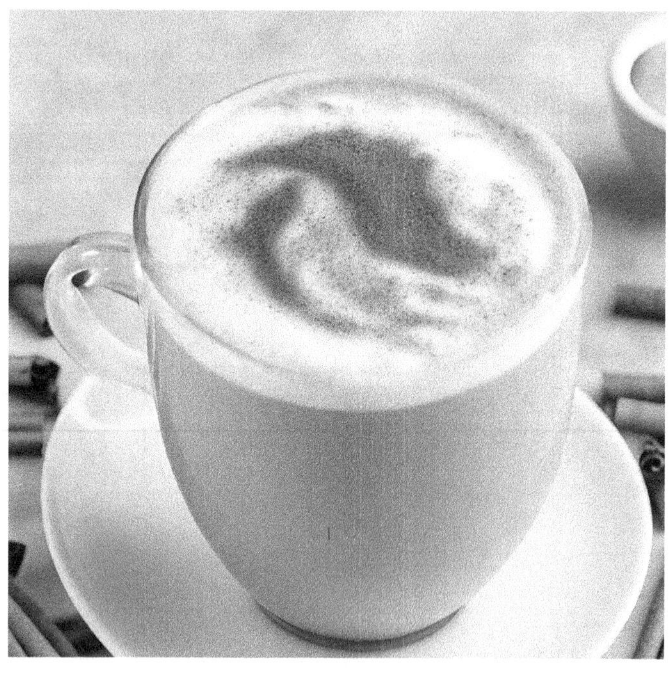

## 14. Beef Liver Pâté with Cucumber Slices

**Ingredients:**

- 1/2 pound beef liver, cleaned and trimmed
- 1/2 cup onion, finely chopped
- 2 cloves garlic, minced
- 1/4 cup extra virgin olive oil
- 1 tablespoon fresh parsley, chopped
- 1 teaspoon sea salt
- 1/2 teaspoon ground black pepper
- 1 large cucumber, sliced

**Instructions:**

1. In a large skillet, heat 2 tablespoons of olive oil over medium heat.
2. Add the onion and garlic, sautéing until soft and translucent, about 5 minutes.
3. Add the beef liver to the skillet and cook until browned on the outside and just cooked through, about 5-7 minutes.
4. Transfer the cooked liver, onions, and garlic to a food processor.
5. Add the remaining olive oil, parsley, sea salt, and black pepper. Blend until smooth and creamy.
6. Serve the pâté with cucumber slices.

**Nutrition Info (Per Serving):**

- Calories: 250
- Protein: 15g
- Carbohydrates: 5g
- Fat: 19g
- Fiber: 1g

**Serves: 4**
**Cooking Time: 20 minutes**

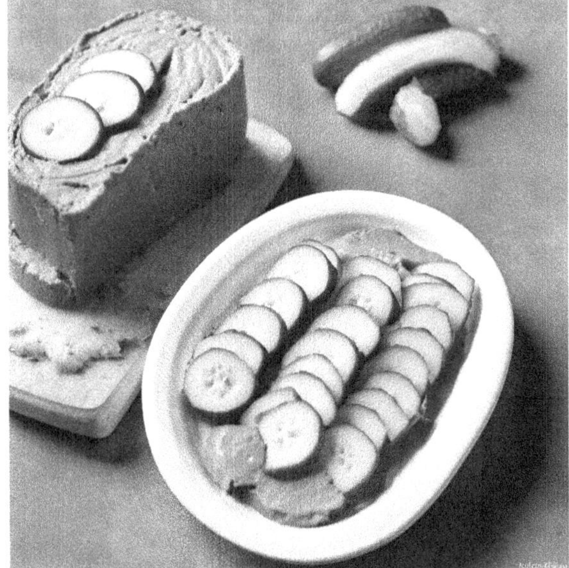

## 15. Celery and Almond Butter

**Ingredients:**

- 4 large celery stalks, cut into 3-inch pieces
- 1/2 cup almond butter
- 1 tablespoon extra virgin olive oil
- 1 teaspoon honey (optional)
- 1/4 teaspoon sea salt

**Instructions:**

1. In a small bowl, mix the almond butter, olive oil, honey, and sea salt until well combined.
2. Spread the almond butter mixture onto the celery pieces.
3. Serve immediately.

**Nutrition Info (Per Serving):**

- Calories: 220
- Protein: 5g
- Carbohydrates: 7g
- Fat: 19g
- Fiber: 4g

**Serves: 2**
**Cooking Time: 5 minutes**

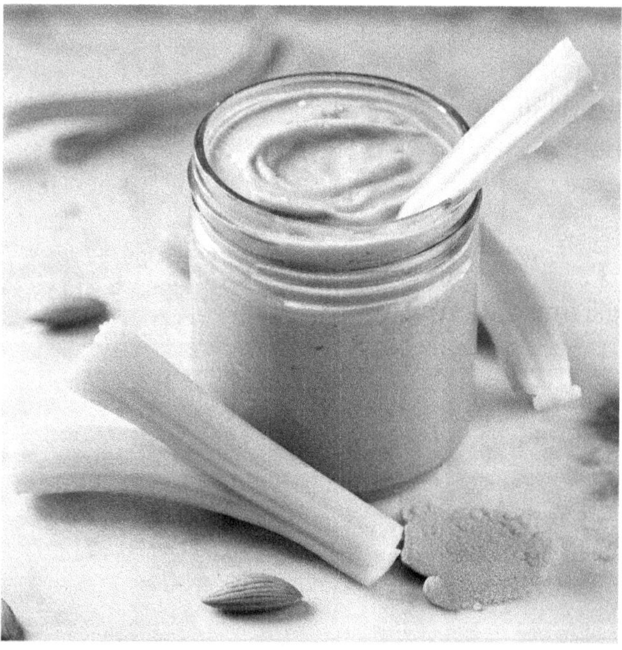

## 16. Baked Coconut Custard

**Ingredients:**

- 1 cup coconut milk
- 3 large eggs
- 1/4 cup honey
- 1 teaspoon vanilla extract
- 1/2 teaspoon ground cinnamon
- 1/4 teaspoon sea salt

**Instructions:**

1. Preheat the oven to 350°F (175°C).
2. In a medium bowl, whisk together the coconut milk, eggs, honey, vanilla extract, cinnamon, and sea salt until well combined.
3. Pour the mixture into ramekins or a small baking dish.
4. Place the ramekins in a baking dish and fill the dish with hot water until it reaches halfway up the sides of the ramekins.
5. Bake in the preheated oven for 30-35 minutes, or until the custard is set.
6. Remove from the oven and let cool before serving.

**Nutrition Info (Per Serving):**

- Calories: 180
- Protein: 5g
- Carbohydrates: 16g
- Fat: 11g
- Fiber: 1g

**Serves: 4**
**Cooking Time: 40 minutes**

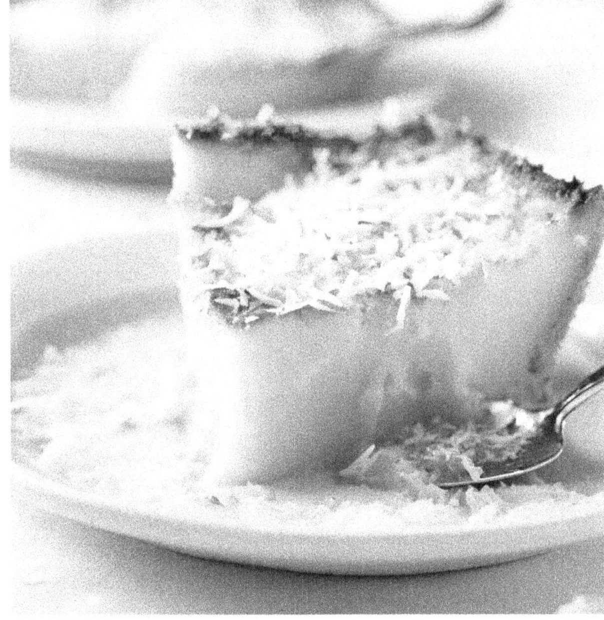

## 17. Collard Greens with Ham

**Ingredients:**

- 4 cups collard greens, washed and chopped
- 1 cup cooked ham, diced
- 1 tablespoon extra virgin olive oil
- 1 onion, finely chopped
- 2 cloves garlic, minced
- 1/4 cup apple cider vinegar
- 1 teaspoon sea salt
- 1/2 teaspoon ground black pepper

**Instructions:**

1. In a large skillet, heat the olive oil over medium heat.
2. Add the onion and garlic, sautéing until translucent, about 5 minutes.
3. Add the diced ham and cook for another 3 minutes.
4. Add the collard greens to the skillet and cook until wilted, about 5-7 minutes.
5. Stir in the apple cider vinegar, sea salt, and black pepper.
6. Cook for another 2-3 minutes, until everything is well combined and heated through.
7. Serve hot.

**Nutrition Info (Per Serving):**

- Calories: 180
- Protein: 10g
- Carbohydrates: 10g
- Fat: 11g
- Fiber: 5g

**Serves: 4**

**Cooking Time: 20 minutes**

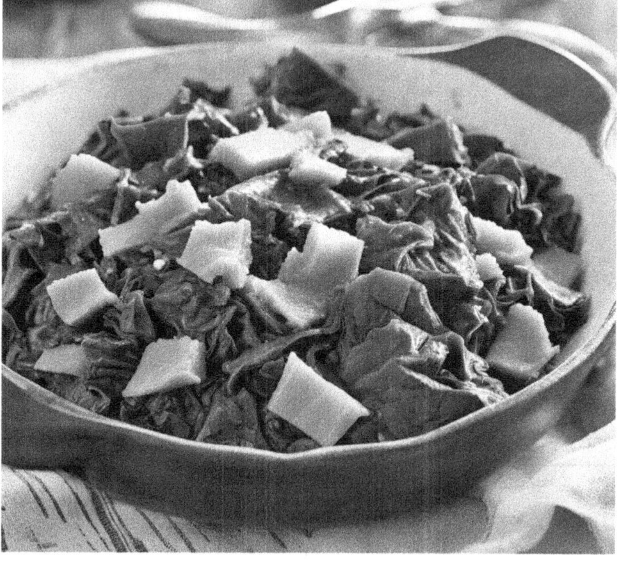

## 18. Beef and Vegetable Breakfast Soup

**Ingredients:**

- 1 pound ground beef
- 1 tablespoon extra virgin olive oil
- 1 large onion, chopped
- 2 cloves garlic, minced
- 4 cups low-sodium beef broth
- 2 cups water
- 2 cups carrots, sliced
- 2 cups celery, sliced
- 2 cups cabbage, chopped
- 1 teaspoon dried thyme
- 1 teaspoon sea salt
- 1/2 teaspoon ground black pepper

**Instructions:**

1. In a large pot, heat the olive oil over medium heat. Add the onion and garlic, sautéing until translucent, about 5 minutes.
2. Add the ground beef, cooking until browned. Drain any excess fat.
3. Pour in the beef broth and water. Add the carrots, celery, cabbage, thyme, sea salt, and black pepper.
4. Bring the soup to a boil, then reduce heat and simmer for 30 minutes, until vegetables are tender.
5. Serve hot.

**Nutrition Info (Per Serving):**

- Calories: 250
- Protein: 20g
- Carbohydrates: 10g
- Fat: 15g
- Fiber: 3g

**Serves: 6**
**Cooking Time: 40 minutes**

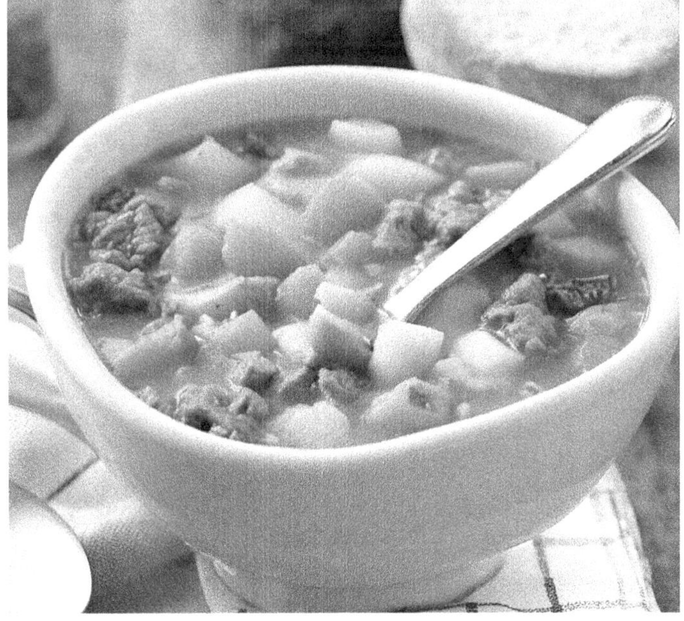

## 19. Herb-Stuffed Mushrooms

**Ingredients:**

- 12 large button mushrooms, stems removed
- 1/4 cup extra virgin olive oil
- 1/2 cup finely chopped onion
- 2 cloves garlic, minced
- 1/4 cup finely chopped fresh parsley
- 1/4 cup finely chopped fresh basil
- 1 teaspoon sea salt
- 1/2 teaspoon ground black pepper

**Instructions:**

1. Preheat the oven to 375°F (190°C).
2. In a skillet, heat 2 tablespoons of olive oil over medium heat. Add the onion and garlic, sautéing until translucent, about 5 minutes.
3. In a bowl, combine the sautéed onion and garlic, parsley, basil, sea salt, and black pepper.
4. Stuff each mushroom cap with the herb mixture.
5. Place the stuffed mushrooms on a baking sheet lined with parchment paper. Drizzle with the remaining olive oil.
6. Bake for 20-25 minutes, until mushrooms are tender.
7. Serve warm.

**Nutrition Info (Per Serving):**

- Calories: 80
- Protein: 2g
- Carbohydrates: 4g
- Fat: 6g
- Fiber: 1g

**Serves: 4**

**Cooking Time: 30 minutes**

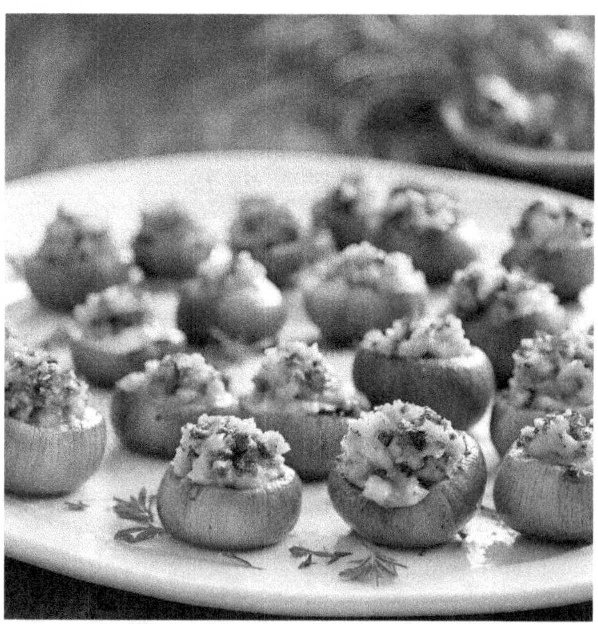

## 20. Broccoli and Chicken Breakfast Casserole

**Ingredients:**

- 2 cups cooked chicken breast, diced
- 2 cups broccoli florets, steamed
- 1/2 cup onion, finely chopped
- 1 cup coconut milk
- 6 large eggs
- 1 teaspoon sea salt
- 1/2 teaspoon ground black pepper
- 1 tablespoon extra virgin olive oil

**Instructions:**

1. Preheat the oven to 350°F (175°C). Grease a 9x13-inch baking dish with olive oil.
2. In a large bowl, combine the chicken, broccoli, and onion. Spread the mixture evenly in the baking dish.
3. In a separate bowl, whisk together the eggs, coconut milk, sea salt, and black pepper. Pour over the chicken and broccoli mixture.
4. Bake for 30-35 minutes, until the casserole is set and golden brown on top.
5. Let cool for a few minutes before serving.

**Nutrition Info (Per Serving):**

- Calories: 220
- Protein: 20g
- Carbohydrates: 6g
- Fat: 14g
- Fiber: 2g

**Serves: 6**
**Cooking Time: 40 minutes**

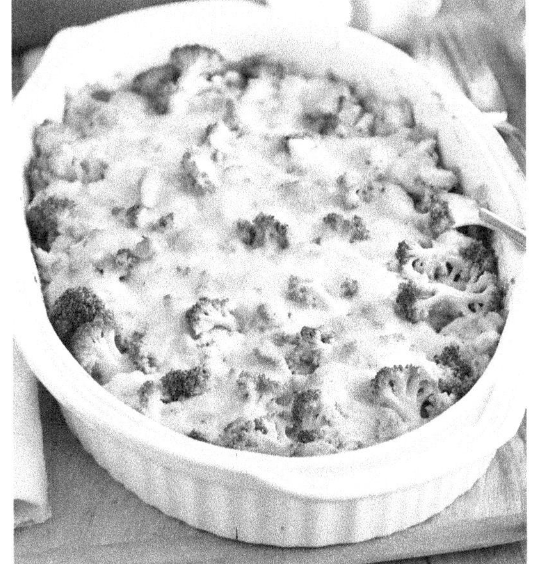

## 21. Coconut Almond Bars

**Ingredients:**

- 1 cup almond flour
- 1 cup unsweetened shredded coconut
- 1/4 cup coconut oil, melted
- 1/4 cup honey
- 1 teaspoon vanilla extract
- 1/4 teaspoon sea salt

**Instructions:**

1. Preheat the oven to 325°F (165°C). Line an 8x8-inch baking dish with parchment paper.
2. In a large bowl, mix together the almond flour, shredded coconut, coconut oil, honey, vanilla extract, and sea salt until well combined.
3. Press the mixture firmly into the prepared baking dish.
4. Bake for 20-25 minutes, until golden brown.
5. Allow to cool completely before cutting into bars.

**Nutrition Info (Per Serving):**

- Calories: 150
- Protein: 3g
- Carbohydrates: 10g
- Fat: 12g
- Fiber: 3g

**Serves: 12**
**Cooking Time: 30 minutes**

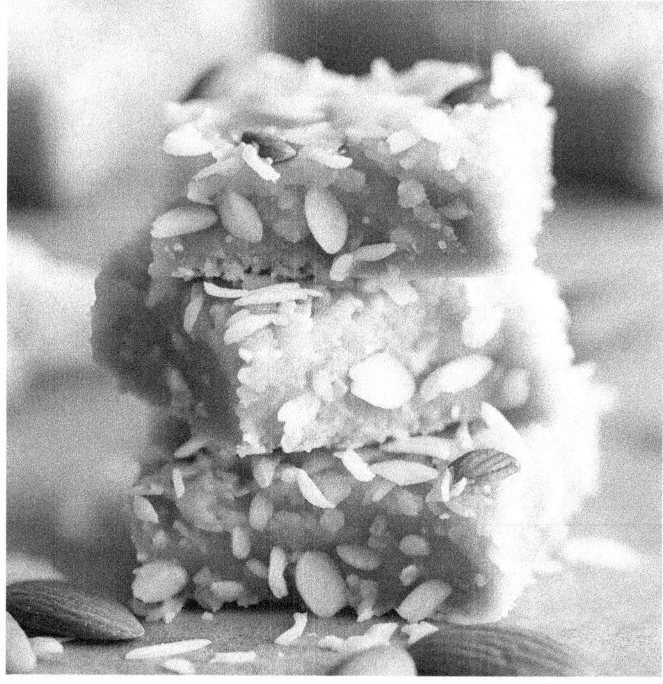

## 22. Sautéed Kale with Poached Eggs

**Ingredients:**

- 4 large eggs
- 1 tablespoon apple cider vinegar
- 1 tablespoon extra virgin olive oil
- 1 large bunch kale, washed and chopped
- 2 cloves garlic, minced
- 1/4 teaspoon sea salt
- 1/4 teaspoon ground black pepper

**Instructions:**

1. Bring a large pot of water to a simmer and add the apple cider vinegar.
2. Crack the eggs into individual small bowls.
3. Stir the simmering water to create a gentle whirlpool and carefully slide each egg into the water. Poach for 3-4 minutes, until the whites are set but the yolks are still runny.
4. Remove the eggs with a slotted spoon and set aside.
5. In a large skillet, heat the olive oil over medium heat. Add the garlic and sauté for 1 minute.
6. Add the kale and cook until wilted, about 5 minutes. Season with sea salt and black pepper.
7. Serve the sautéed kale topped with poached eggs.

**Nutrition Info (Per Serving):**

- Calories: 180
- Protein: 10g
- Carbohydrates: 8g
- Fat: 12g
- Fiber: 2g

**Serves: 2**

**Cooking Time: 15 minutes**

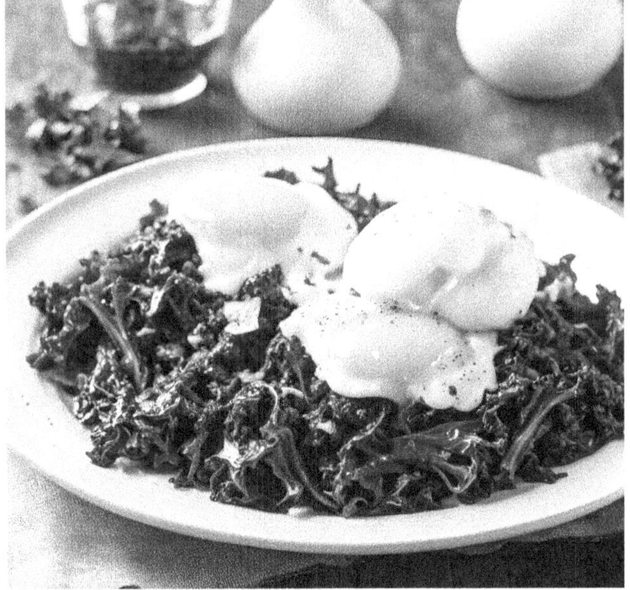

## 23. Almond Butter Banana Smoothie

**Ingredients:**

- 1 ripe banana
- 1/4 cup almond butter
- 1 cup unsweetened almond milk
- 1 teaspoon vanilla extract
- 1/4 teaspoon ground cinnamon
- 1/2 cup ice cubes

**Instructions:**

1. Combine all ingredients in a blender.
2. Blend on high until smooth and creamy.
3. Pour into glasses and serve immediately.

Nutrition Info (Per Serving):

- Calories: 250
- Protein: 5g
- Carbohydrates: 25g
- Fat: 16g
- Fiber: 4g

**Serves: 2**

**Cooking Time: 5 minutes**

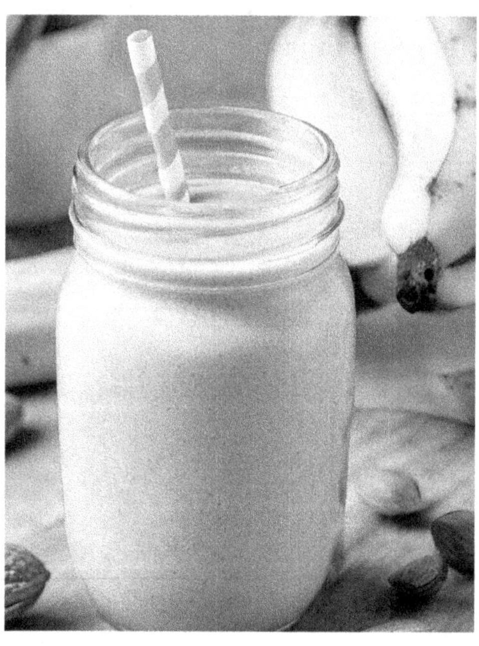

## 24. Pumpkin Seed Muesli

**Ingredients:**

- 1 cup unsweetened coconut flakes
- 1/2 cup pumpkin seeds
- 1/4 cup chia seeds
- 1/4 cup flaxseeds
- 1/4 cup dried cranberries (unsweetened)
- 1 teaspoon ground cinnamon
- 1 cup unsweetened almond milk

**Instructions:**

1. In a large bowl, combine the coconut flakes, pumpkin seeds, chia seeds, flaxseeds, dried cranberries, and cinnamon.
2. Serve 1/2 cup of the muesli mixture with 1/2 cup of almond milk per serving.

**Nutrition Info (Per Serving):**

- Calories: 220
- Protein: 6g
- Carbohydrates: 12g
- Fat: 16g
- Fiber: 7g

**Serves: 4**
**Cooking Time: 5 minutes**

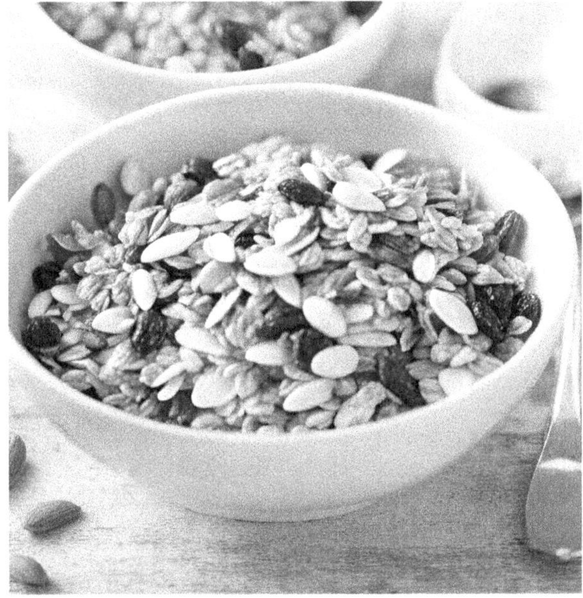

## 25. Kale and Olive Oil Smoothie

**Ingredients:**

- 1 cup kale leaves, washed and chopped
- 1/2 avocado
- 1/2 cup unsweetened almond milk
- 1 tablespoon extra virgin olive oil
- 1 teaspoon honey
- 1/2 cup ice cubes

**Instructions:**

1. Combine all ingredients in a blender.
2. Blend on high until smooth and creamy.
3. Pour into glasses and serve immediately.

**Nutrition Info (Per Serving):**

- Calories: 200
- Protein: 2g
- Carbohydrates: 10g
- Fat: 18g
- Fiber: 5g

**Serves: 2**

**Cooking Time: 5 minutes**

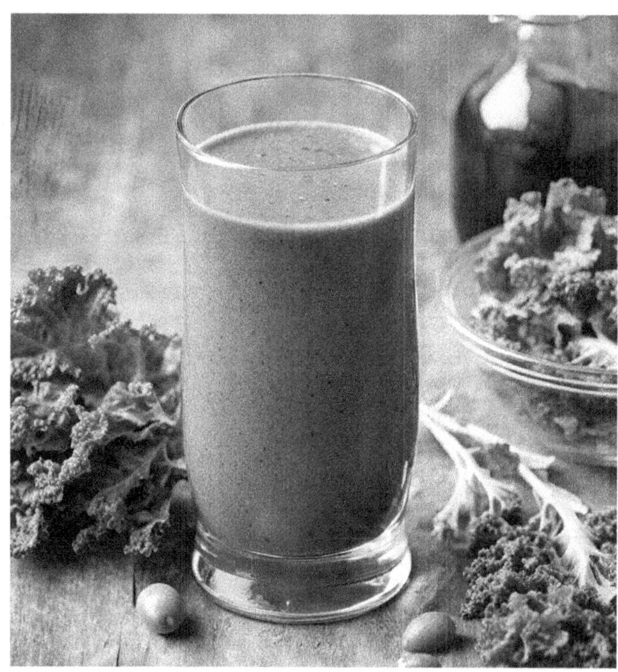

## 26. Flaxseed Porridge

**Ingredients:**

- 1/4 cup ground flaxseeds
- 1/4 cup unsweetened almond milk
- 1 tablespoon chia seeds
- 1 tablespoon almond butter
- 1 teaspoon honey
- 1/2 teaspoon ground cinnamon

**Instructions:**

1. In a small saucepan, combine the ground flaxseeds, almond milk, chia seeds, almond butter, honey, and cinnamon.
2. Cook over medium heat, stirring constantly, until thickened, about 3-5 minutes.
3. Serve warm.

**Nutrition Info (Per Serving):**

- Calories: 250
- Protein: 7g
- Carbohydrates: 15g
- Fat: 18g
- Fiber: 12g

**Serves: 1**
**Cooking Time: 5 minutes**

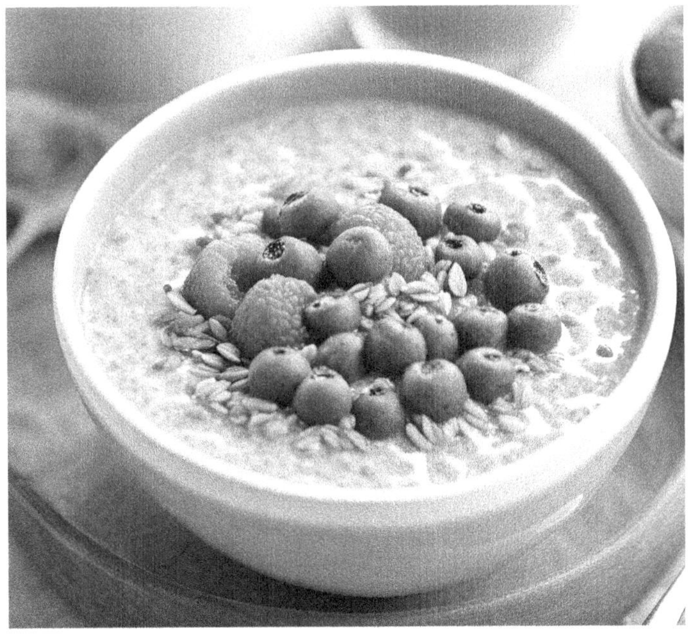

## 27. Almond Flour Pancakes

**Ingredients:**

- 1 cup almond flour
- 1/4 cup coconut flour
- 1/2 teaspoon baking soda
- 3 large eggs
- 1/4 cup unsweetened almond milk
- 1 tablespoon honey
- 1 teaspoon vanilla extract
- 1/4 cup extra virgin olive oil (for cooking)

**Instructions:**

1. In a large bowl, whisk together the almond flour, coconut flour, and baking soda.
2. In a separate bowl, beat the eggs and then add the almond milk, honey, and vanilla extract.
3. Combine the wet and dry ingredients, mixing until smooth.
4. Heat the olive oil in a large skillet over medium heat.
5. Pour 1/4 cup of batter onto the skillet for each pancake. Cook until bubbles form on the surface, then flip and cook until golden brown.
6. Serve warm.

**Nutrition Info (Per Serving):**

- Calories: 180
- Protein: 6g
- Carbohydrates: 8g
- Fat: 14g
- Fiber: 3g

Serves: 4

Cooking Time: 20 minutes

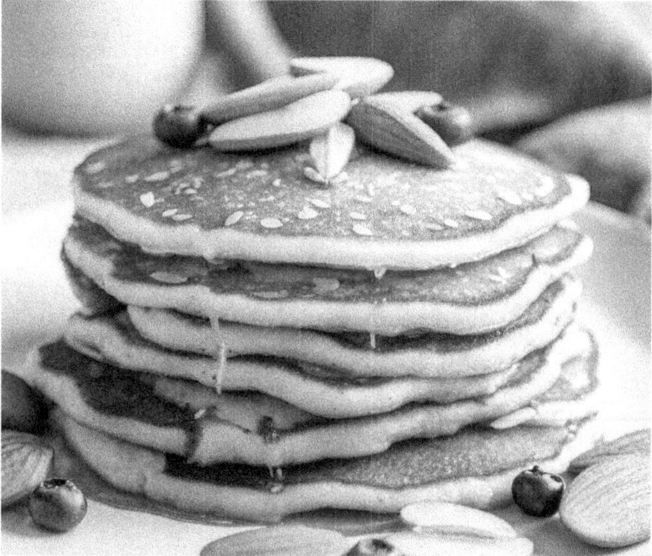

# Vegetables

## 1. Kale Caesar Salad

**Ingredients:**

- 6 cups kale, washed and chopped
- 1/4 cup extra virgin olive oil
- 2 tablespoons lemon juice
- 1 teaspoon Dijon mustard
- 2 cloves garlic, minced
- 1/4 cup grated Parmesan cheese (optional, if tolerable)
- 1/4 cup sunflower seeds
- 1/4 teaspoon sea salt
- 1/4 teaspoon ground black pepper

**Instructions:**

1. In a large bowl, combine the olive oil, lemon juice, Dijon mustard, and minced garlic. Whisk until well blended.
2. Add the chopped kale to the bowl and toss to coat with the dressing.
3. Sprinkle with Parmesan cheese (if using), sunflower seeds, sea salt, and black pepper.
4. Toss again to combine.
5. Serve immediately.

**Nutrition Info (Per Serving):**

- Calories: 180
- Protein: 5g
- Carbohydrates: 10g
- Fat: 14g
- Fiber: 4g

**Serves: 4**
**Cooking Time: 15 minutes**

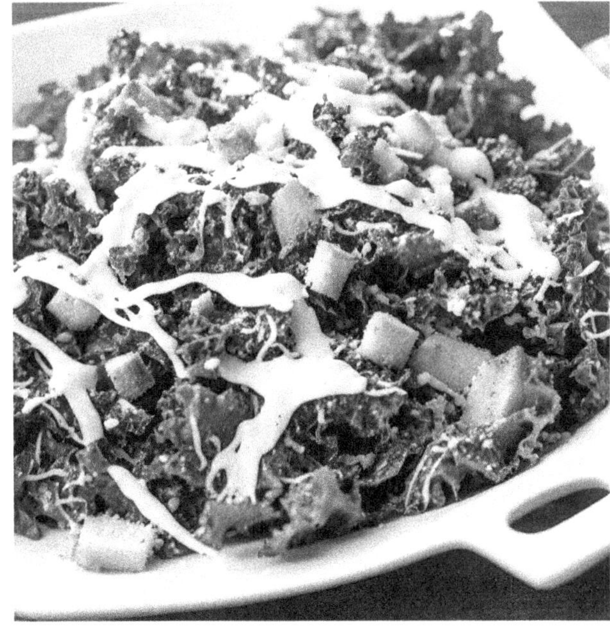

## 2. Collard Greens with Garlic

**Ingredients:**

- 6 cups collard greens, washed and chopped
- 3 tablespoons extra virgin olive oil
- 4 cloves garlic, minced
- 1/4 cup apple cider vinegar
- 1 teaspoon sea salt
- 1/2 teaspoon ground black pepper

**Instructions:**

1. In a large skillet, heat the olive oil over medium heat.
2. Add the minced garlic and sauté for 1-2 minutes, until fragrant.
3. Add the chopped collard greens to the skillet and sauté for 5-7 minutes, until wilted.
4. Stir in the apple cider vinegar, sea salt, and black pepper.
5. Cook for another 2-3 minutes, until the greens are tender.
6. Serve hot.

**Nutrition Info (Per Serving):**

- Calories: 140
- Protein: 3g
- Carbohydrates: 10g
- Fat: 11g
- Fiber: 5g

**Serves: 4**
**Cooking Time: 15 minutes**

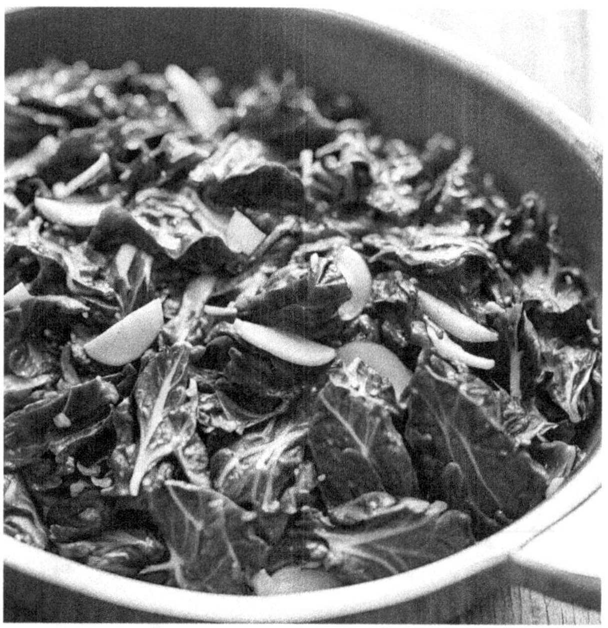

### 3. Swiss Chard and Pine Nuts

**Ingredients:**

- 6 cups Swiss chard, washed and chopped
- 2 tablespoons extra virgin olive oil
- 1/4 cup pine nuts
- 1/2 cup onion, finely chopped
- 2 cloves garlic, minced
- 1/4 teaspoon sea salt
- 1/4 teaspoon ground black pepper

**Instructions:**

1. In a large skillet, heat the olive oil over medium heat.
2. Add the pine nuts and toast until golden brown, about 3 minutes. Remove from the skillet and set aside.
3. In the same skillet, add the onion and garlic. Sauté until translucent, about 5 minutes.
4. Add the Swiss chard to the skillet and cook until wilted, about 5-7 minutes.
5. Season with sea salt and black pepper.
6. Stir in the toasted pine nuts.
7. Serve hot.

**Nutrition Info (Per Serving):**

- Calories: 170
- Protein: 4g
- Carbohydrates: 10g
- Fat: 14g
- Fiber: 3g

**Serves: 4**

**Cooking Time: 20 minutes**

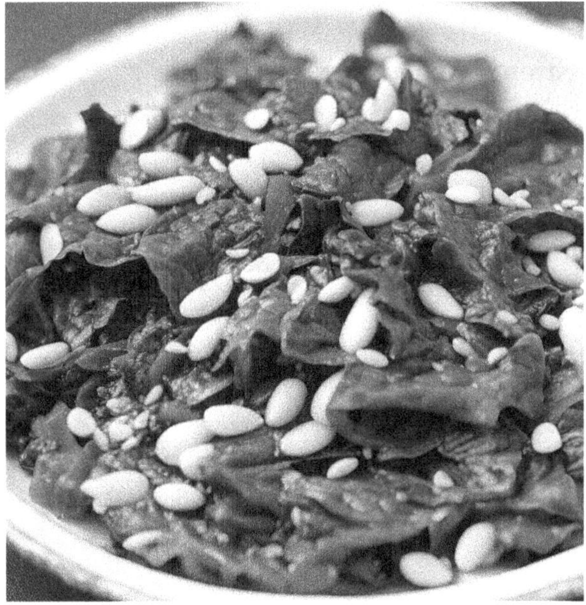

## 4. Mustard Greens Spicy Stir Fry

**Ingredients:**

- 6 cups mustard greens, washed and chopped
- 2 tablespoons extra virgin olive oil
- 1 tablespoon fresh ginger, grated
- 2 cloves garlic, minced
- 1/2 teaspoon red pepper flakes
- 2 tablespoons coconut aminos
- 1 teaspoon sesame oil
- 1 teaspoon sea salt
- 1/2 teaspoon ground black pepper

**Instructions:**

1. In a large skillet, heat the olive oil over medium heat.
2. Add the grated ginger, minced garlic, and red pepper flakes. Sauté for 2-3 minutes until fragrant.
3. Add the chopped mustard greens to the skillet and stir-fry for 5-7 minutes, until wilted.
4. Stir in the coconut aminos and sesame oil.
5. Season with sea salt and black pepper.
6. Cook for another 2-3 minutes, until the greens are tender and the flavors are well combined.
7. Serve hot.

**Nutrition Info (Per Serving):**

- Calories: 130
- Protein: 3g
- Carbohydrates: 8g
- Fat: 11g
- Fiber: 4g

**Serves: 4**

**Cooking Time: 15 minutes**

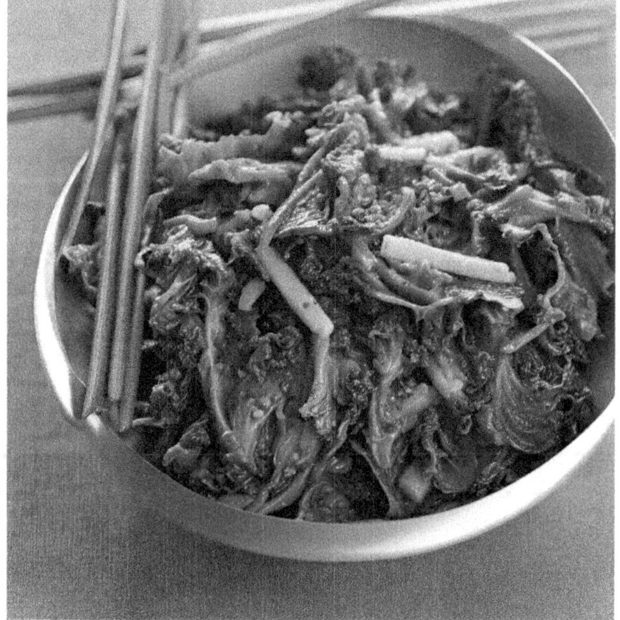

## 5. Broccoli Almond Salad

**Ingredients:**

- 4 cups broccoli florets, blanched
- 1/2 cup sliced almonds, toasted
- 1/4 cup red onion, finely chopped
- 1/4 cup raisins
- 1/4 cup extra virgin olive oil
- 2 tablespoons apple cider vinegar
- 1 tablespoon honey
- 1 teaspoon Dijon mustard
- 1/2 teaspoon sea salt
- 1/4 teaspoon ground black pepper

**Instructions:**

1. In a large bowl, combine the blanched broccoli, toasted almonds, red onion, and raisins.
2. In a small bowl, whisk together the olive oil, apple cider vinegar, honey, Dijon mustard, sea salt, and black pepper.
3. Pour the dressing over the broccoli mixture and toss to coat.
4. Serve immediately or chill for 30 minutes to let the flavors meld.

**Nutrition Info (Per Serving):**

- Calories: 180
- Protein: 4g
- Carbohydrates: 12g
- Fat: 14g
- Fiber: 4g

**Serves: 4**
**Cooking Time: 15 minutes**

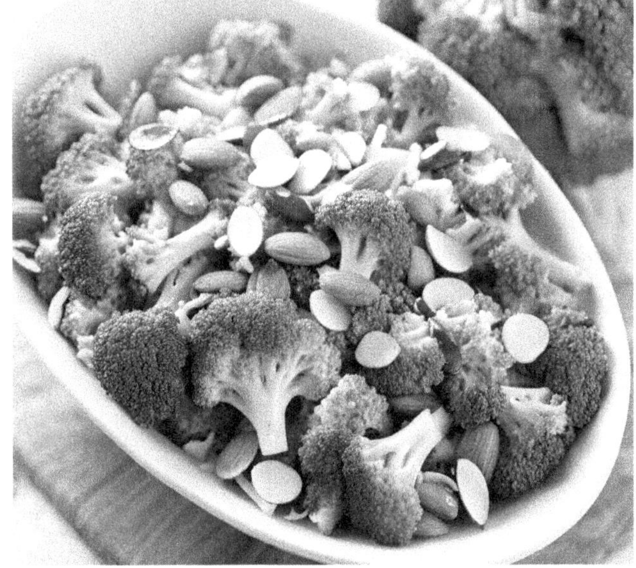

**6. Cauliflower Rice Pilaf**
**Ingredients:**

- 1 large head cauliflower, grated into rice-sized pieces
- 1/4 cup extra virgin olive oil
- 1/2 cup onion, finely chopped
- 2 cloves garlic, minced
- 1/4 cup sliced almonds, toasted
- 1/4 cup raisins
- 1 teaspoon ground turmeric
- 1 teaspoon ground cumin
- 1 teaspoon sea salt
- 1/4 teaspoon ground black pepper
- 1/4 cup fresh parsley, chopped

**Instructions:**

1. In a large skillet, heat the olive oil over medium heat.
2. Add the onion and garlic, sautéing until translucent, about 5 minutes.
3. Add the grated cauliflower, turmeric, cumin, sea salt, and black pepper. Cook for 5-7 minutes, until the cauliflower is tender.
4. Stir in the toasted almonds and raisins.
5. Remove from heat and stir in the fresh parsley.
6. Serve hot.

**Nutrition Info (Per Serving):**

- Calories: 160
- Protein: 4g
- Carbohydrates: 12g
- Fat: 12g
- Fiber: 5g

**Serves: 4**
**Cooking Time: 15 minutes**

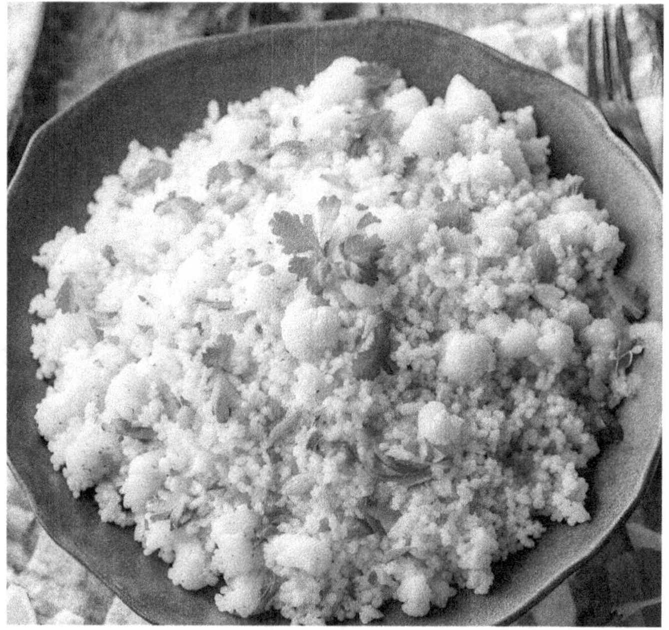

# 7. Korean Kimchi

**Ingredients:**

- 1 medium napa cabbage, chopped
- 2 tablespoons sea salt
- 1/4 cup grated carrot
- 1/4 cup grated daikon radish
- 4 green onions, chopped
- 2 tablespoons fresh ginger, grated
- 4 cloves garlic, minced
- 2 tablespoons coconut aminos
- 1 tablespoon fish sauce (optional)
- 1 teaspoon red pepper flakes

**Instructions:**

1. In a large bowl, toss the chopped cabbage with sea salt and let sit for 1-2 hours to draw out moisture. Rinse and drain.
2. In a separate bowl, mix the grated carrot, daikon radish, green onions, ginger, garlic, coconut aminos, fish sauce (if using), and red pepper flakes.
3. Add the drained cabbage to the mixture and toss to combine.
4. Pack the mixture tightly into a clean jar, pressing down to remove air pockets.
5. Let ferment at room temperature for 3-7 days, tasting until desired tanginess is achieved.
6. Store in the refrigerator.

**Nutrition Info (Per Serving):**

- Calories: 40
- Protein: 2g
- Carbohydrates: 8g
- Fat: 0g
- Fiber: 3g

**Serves: 8**

**Cooking Time: 30 minutes (plus fermentation time)**

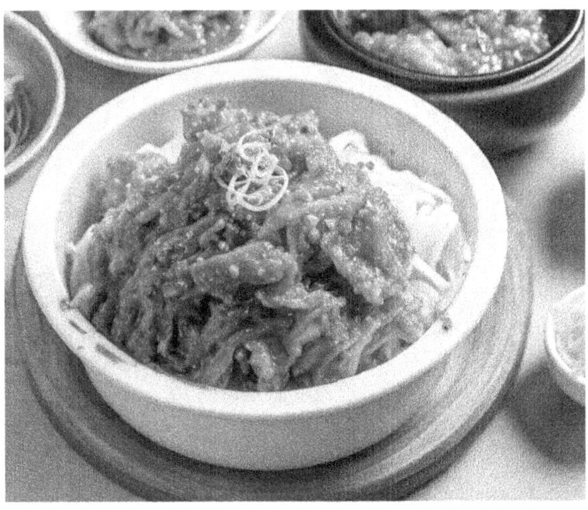

## 8. Bok Choy and Shiitake Mushroom Stir-Fry

**Ingredients:**

- 4 cups bok choy, washed and chopped
- 2 cups shiitake mushrooms, sliced
- 2 tablespoons extra virgin olive oil
- 1/4 cup onion, finely chopped
- 2 cloves garlic, minced
- 2 tablespoons coconut aminos
- 1 teaspoon sesame oil
- 1/2 teaspoon sea salt
- 1/4 teaspoon ground black pepper

**Instructions:**

1. In a large skillet, heat the olive oil over medium heat.
2. Add the onion and garlic, sautéing until translucent, about 5 minutes.
3. Add the shiitake mushrooms and cook for 3-4 minutes, until softened.
4. Add the bok choy, coconut aminos, sesame oil, sea salt, and black pepper. Stir-fry for 5-7 minutes, until the bok choy is tender.
5. Serve hot.

**Nutrition Info (Per Serving):**

- Calories: 120
- Protein: 3g
- Carbohydrates: 8g
- Fat: 10g
- Fiber: 3g

**Serves: 4**
**Cooking Time: 15 minutes**

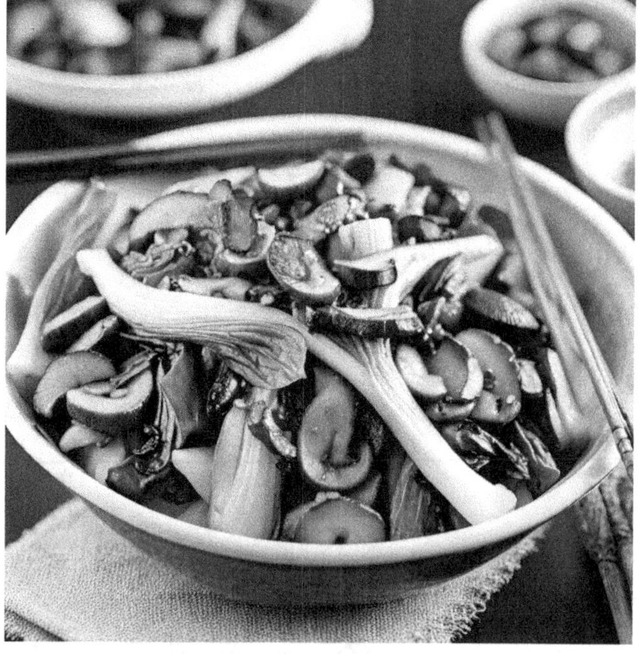

## 9. Roasted Garlic Spread

**Ingredients:**

- 2 heads garlic
- 2 tablespoons extra virgin olive oil
- 1/2 teaspoon sea salt
- 1/4 teaspoon ground black pepper
- 1 teaspoon fresh thyme, chopped

**Instructions:**

1. Preheat the oven to 400°F (200°C).
2. Cut the tops off the garlic heads to expose the cloves. Place them on a piece of aluminum foil.
3. Drizzle the garlic with olive oil and sprinkle with sea salt and black pepper. Wrap the foil around the garlic to form a packet.
4. Roast in the preheated oven for 30-35 minutes, until the garlic is soft and caramelized.
5. Let cool slightly, then squeeze the roasted garlic cloves out of their skins into a bowl.
6. Mash with a fork and stir in the fresh thyme.
7. Serve as a spread on vegetables or low-lectin crackers.

**Nutrition Info (Per Serving):**

- Calories: 80
- Protein: 1g
- Carbohydrates: 9g
- Fat: 5g
- Fiber: 1g

Serves: 4

Cooking Time: 40 minutes

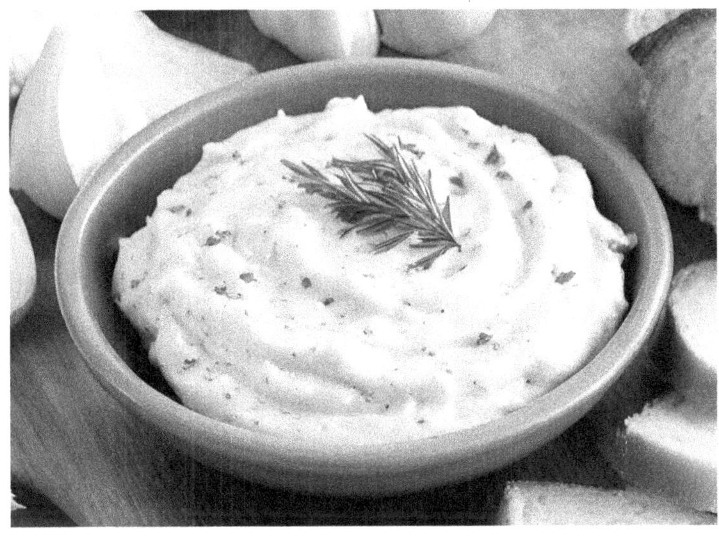

## 10. Leek and Herb Frittata

**Ingredients:**

- 1 tablespoon extra virgin olive oil
- 1 large leek, washed and thinly sliced
- 8 large eggs
- 1/4 cup coconut milk
- 1/4 cup fresh parsley, chopped
- 1/4 cup fresh chives, chopped
- 1 teaspoon sea salt
- 1/2 teaspoon ground black pepper

**Instructions:**

1. Preheat the oven to 350°F (175°C).
2. In a large oven-safe skillet, heat the olive oil over medium heat. Add the sliced leek and sauté until soft, about 5 minutes.
3. In a bowl, whisk together the eggs, coconut milk, parsley, chives, sea salt, and black pepper.
4. Pour the egg mixture over the leeks in the skillet.
5. Cook on the stovetop over medium heat for 5 minutes, until the edges begin to set.
6. Transfer the skillet to the preheated oven and bake for 15-20 minutes, until the frittata is fully set and golden brown.
7. Let cool slightly before slicing and serving.

**Nutrition Info (Per Serving):**

- Calories: 160
- Protein: 10g
- Carbohydrates: 5g
- Fat: 12g
- Fiber: 1g

**Serves: 4**

**Cooking Time: 30 minutes**

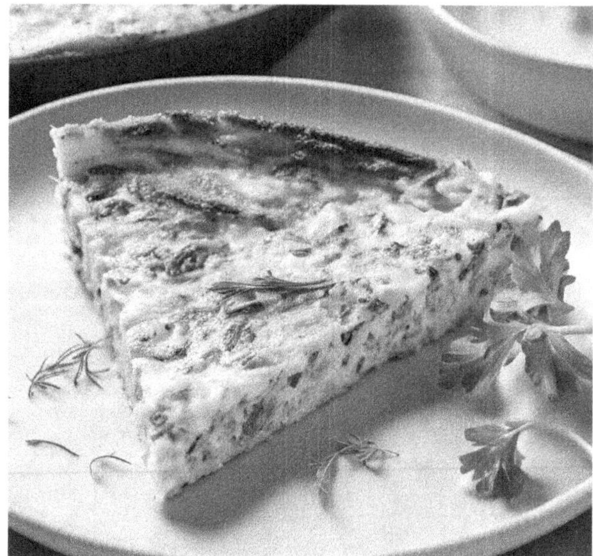

## 11. Scallion Pancakes

**Ingredients:**

- 1 cup almond flour
- 1/4 cup coconut flour
- 1/2 teaspoon baking soda
- 1/2 teaspoon sea salt
- 3 large eggs
- 1/4 cup unsweetened almond milk
- 1/4 cup scallions, finely chopped
- 1 tablespoon extra virgin olive oil (for cooking)

**Instructions:**

1. In a large bowl, whisk together the almond flour, coconut flour, baking soda, and sea salt.
2. In a separate bowl, beat the eggs and then add the almond milk.
3. Combine the wet and dry ingredients, mixing until smooth. Fold in the chopped scallions.
4. Heat the olive oil in a large skillet over medium heat.
5. Pour 1/4 cup of batter onto the skillet for each pancake. Cook until bubbles form on the surface, then flip and cook until golden brown.
6. Serve warm.

**Nutrition Info (Per Serving):**

- Calories: 180
- Protein: 7g
- Carbohydrates: 8g
- Fat: 14g
- Fiber: 3g

**Serves: 4**
**Cooking Time: 20 minutes**

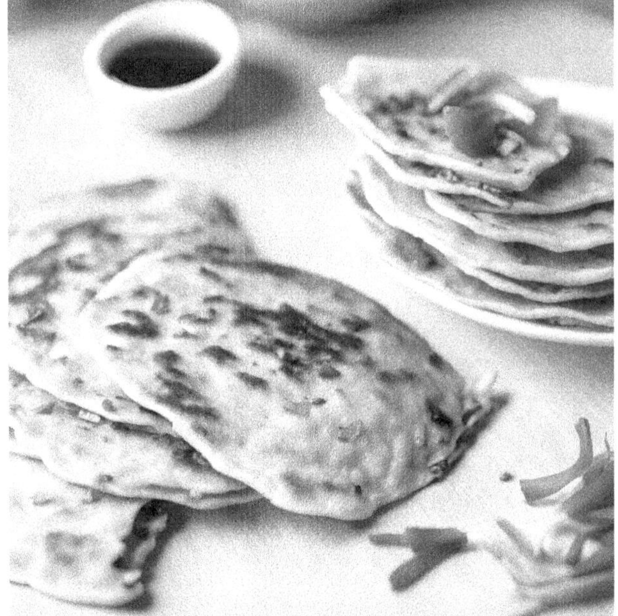

## 12. Garlic and Herb Roasted Shallots

**Ingredients:**

- 1 pound shallots, peeled and halved
- 3 tablespoons extra virgin olive oil
- 4 cloves garlic, minced
- 1 tablespoon fresh thyme, chopped
- 1 tablespoon fresh rosemary, chopped
- 1/2 teaspoon sea salt
- 1/4 teaspoon ground black pepper

**Instructions:**

1. Preheat the oven to 400°F (200°C).
2. In a large bowl, toss the shallots with olive oil, garlic, thyme, rosemary, sea salt, and black pepper.
3. Spread the shallots in a single layer on a baking sheet.
4. Roast in the preheated oven for 25-30 minutes, until the shallots are caramelized and tender.
5. Serve warm.

**Nutrition Info (Per Serving):**

- Calories: 120
- Protein: 2g
- Carbohydrates: 15g
- Fat: 7g
- Fiber: 3g

**Serves: 4**
**Cooking Time: 35 minutes**

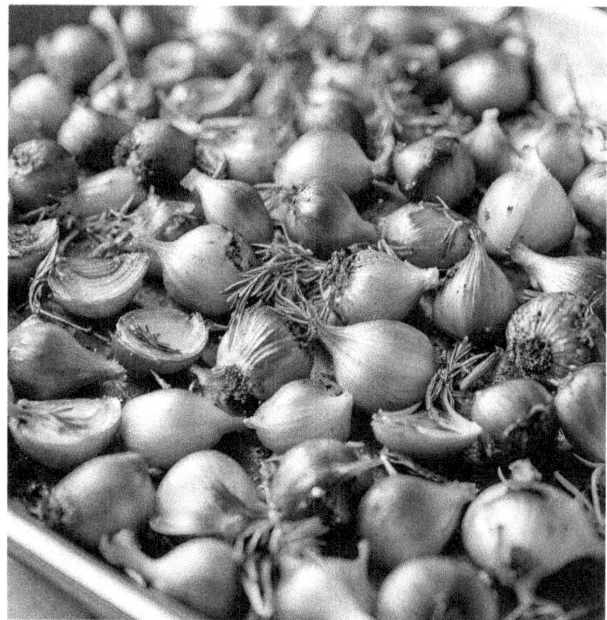

## 13. Beet and Goat Cheese Salad

**Ingredients:**

- 4 medium beets, roasted and sliced
- 4 cups mixed greens (such as arugula, spinach, and kale)
- 1/4 cup goat cheese, crumbled
- 1/4 cup walnuts, toasted and chopped
- 1/4 cup extra virgin olive oil
- 2 tablespoons balsamic vinegar
- 1 teaspoon honey
- 1/2 teaspoon sea salt
- 1/4 teaspoon ground black pepper

**Instructions:**

1. In a small bowl, whisk together the olive oil, balsamic vinegar, honey, sea salt, and black pepper.
2. In a large bowl, combine the mixed greens, roasted beets, goat cheese, and toasted walnuts.
3. Drizzle the dressing over the salad and toss gently to combine.
4. Serve immediately.

**Nutrition Info (Per Serving):**

- Calories: 200
- Protein: 5g
- Carbohydrates: 15g
- Fat: 15g
- Fiber: 4g

**Serves: 4**

**Cooking Time: 45 minutes (including roasting time)**

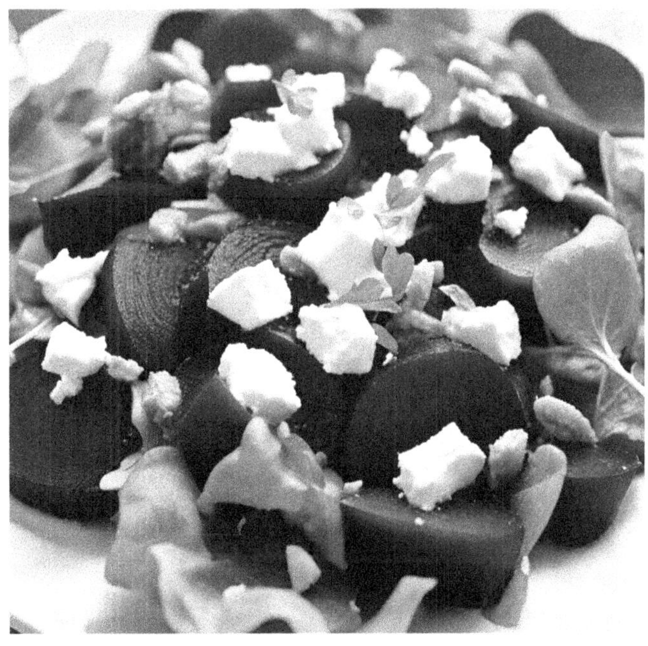

## 14. Turnip Au Gratin

**Ingredients:**

- 4 medium turnips, peeled and thinly sliced
- 1/2 cup coconut milk
- 1/4 cup nutritional yeast
- 2 cloves garlic, minced
- 1 tablespoon fresh thyme, chopped
- 1 teaspoon sea salt
- 1/2 teaspoon ground black pepper
- 2 tablespoons extra virgin olive oil

**Instructions:**

1. Preheat the oven to 375°F (190°C).
2. In a small bowl, mix together the coconut milk, nutritional yeast, garlic, thyme, sea salt, and black pepper.
3. Layer the sliced turnips in a greased baking dish.
4. Pour the coconut milk mixture over the turnips.
5. Drizzle with olive oil.
6. Bake in the preheated oven for 35-40 minutes, until the turnips are tender and the top is golden brown.
7. Serve hot.

**Nutrition Info (Per Serving):**

- Calories: 160
- Protein: 3g
- Carbohydrates: 12g
- Fat: 12g
- Fiber: 4g

**Serves: 4**
**Cooking Time: 45 minutes**

## 15. Radish Raita

**Ingredients:**

- 1 cup radishes, grated
- 1 cup coconut yogurt
- 2 tablespoons fresh mint, chopped
- 1 tablespoon fresh dill, chopped
- 1 teaspoon cumin seeds, toasted and ground
- 1/2 teaspoon sea salt
- 1/4 teaspoon ground black pepper

**Instructions:**

1. In a medium bowl, combine the grated radishes, coconut yogurt, mint, dill, ground cumin, sea salt, and black pepper.
2. Mix well until all ingredients are evenly distributed.
3. Chill for 30 minutes before serving to let the flavors meld.
4. Serve cold.

**Nutrition Info (Per Serving):**

- Calories: 80
- Protein: 2g
- Carbohydrates: 6g
- Fat: 5g
- Fiber: 2g

**Serves: 4**

**Cooking Time: 10 minutes (plus chilling time)**

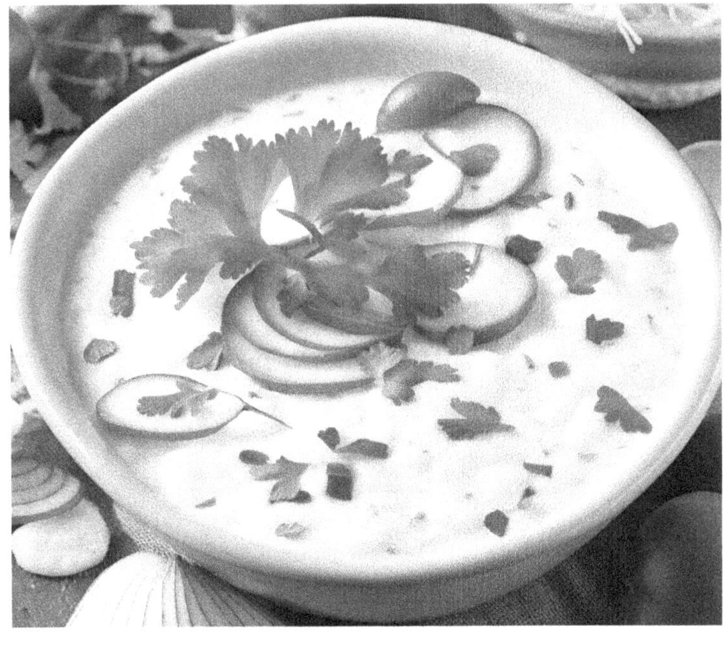

## 16. Ethiopian Collard Greens (Gomen)

**Ingredients:**

- 1 large bunch collard greens, washed and chopped
- 1/4 cup extra virgin olive oil
- 1 large onion, finely chopped
- 4 cloves garlic, minced
- 1 teaspoon ground ginger
- 1 teaspoon ground turmeric
- 1 teaspoon ground cardamom
- 1 teaspoon sea salt
- 1/2 teaspoon ground black pepper
- 1/4 cup water

**Instructions:**

1. In a large pot, heat the olive oil over medium heat.
2. Add the onion and garlic, sautéing until translucent, about 5 minutes.
3. Add the ground ginger, turmeric, and cardamom, cooking for another 2 minutes.
4. Add the collard greens, sea salt, black pepper, and water. Stir well to combine.
5. Cover and cook for 15-20 minutes, until the collard greens are tender.
6. Serve hot.

**Nutrition Info (Per Serving):**

- Calories: 140
- Protein: 3g
- Carbohydrates: 10g
- Fat: 11g
- Fiber: 4g

**Serves: 4**

**Cooking Time: 30 minutes**

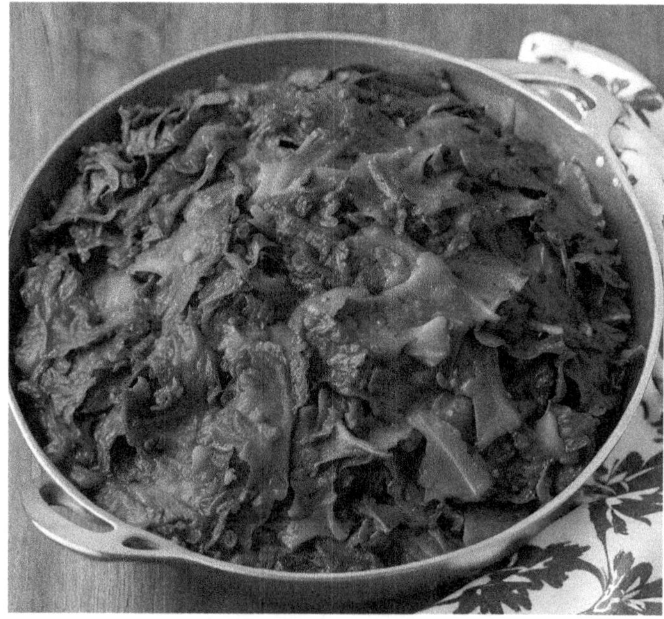

# 17. Indian Spiced Cauliflower (Gobi Masala)

**Ingredients:**

- 1 large head cauliflower, cut into florets
- 3 tablespoons extra virgin olive oil
- 1 large onion, finely chopped
- 2 cloves garlic, minced
- 1 tablespoon fresh ginger, grated
- 1 teaspoon ground cumin
- 1 teaspoon ground coriander
- 1/2 teaspoon ground turmeric
- 1/2 teaspoon ground cumin
- 1/4 teaspoon ground black pepper
- 1/4 cup coconut milk
- 1/4 cup fresh cilantro, chopped

**Instructions:**

1. In a large skillet, heat the olive oil over medium heat.
2. Add the onion, garlic, and ginger, sautéing until translucent, about 5 minutes.
3. Add the ground cumin, coriander, turmeric, and black pepper, cooking for another 2 minutes.
4. Add the cauliflower florets, stirring to coat with the spices.
5. Pour in the coconut milk and stir well to combine.
6. Cover and cook for 10-15 minutes, until the cauliflower is tender.
7. Garnish with fresh cilantro before serving.
8. Serve hot.

**Nutrition Info (Per Serving):**

- Calories: 180
- Protein: 4g
- Carbohydrates: 12g
- Fat: 14g
- Fiber: 5g

**Serves: 4**
**Cooking Time: 25 minutes**

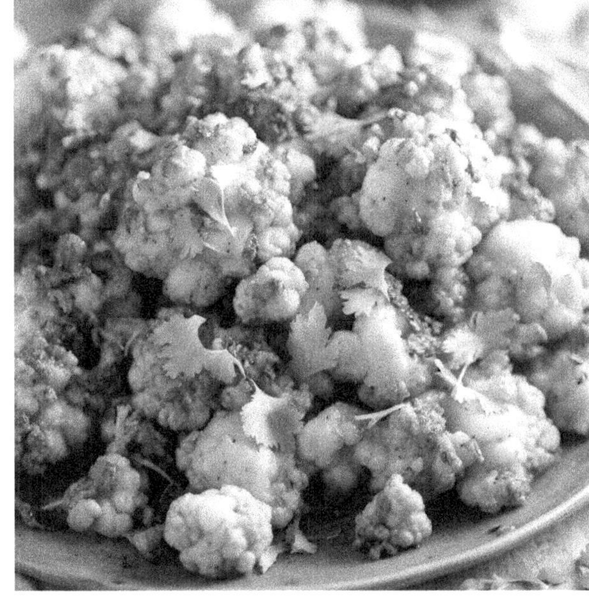

## 18. Japanese Daikon Radish Salad

**Ingredients:**

- 2 cups daikon radish, julienned
- 1 cup carrot, julienned
- 1/4 cup rice vinegar
- 1 tablespoon sesame oil
- 1 tablespoon honey
- 1 tablespoon sesame seeds
- 1 teaspoon grated fresh ginger
- 1/4 teaspoon sea salt
- 1/4 teaspoon ground black pepper
- 2 tablespoons fresh cilantro, chopped

**Instructions:**

1. In a large bowl, combine the julienned daikon radish and carrot.
2. In a small bowl, whisk together the rice vinegar, sesame oil, honey, sesame seeds, grated ginger, sea salt, and black pepper.
3. Pour the dressing over the daikon and carrot, tossing to coat.
4. Garnish with fresh cilantro.
5. Serve immediately or chill for 30 minutes to let the flavors meld.

**Nutrition Info (Per Serving):**

- Calories: 80
- Protein: 1g
- Carbohydrates: 10g
- Fat: 4g
- Fiber: 3g

**Serves: 4**
**Cooking Time: 15 minutes**

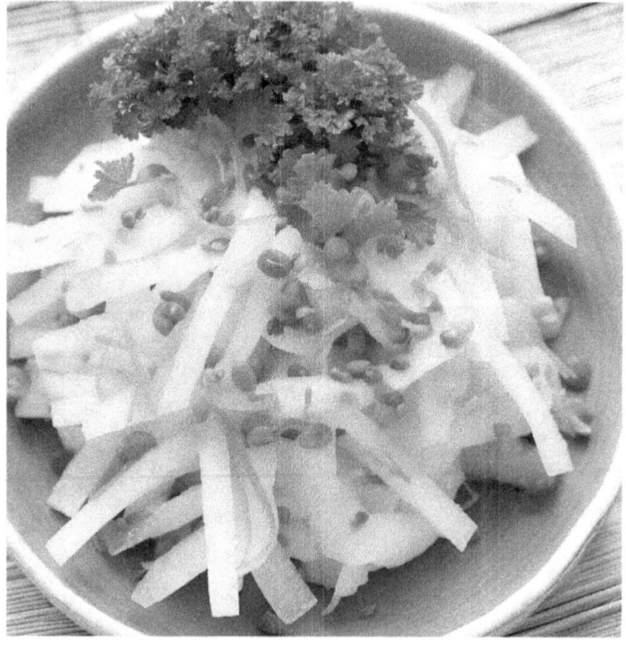

## 19. Thai Coconut Soup with Bok Choy

**Ingredients:**

- 1 tablespoon extra virgin olive oil
- 1 large onion, finely chopped
- 2 cloves garlic, minced
- 1 tablespoon fresh ginger, grated
- 4 cups low-sodium vegetable broth
- 1 can (14 oz) coconut milk
- 2 cups bok choy, chopped
- 1 cup mushrooms, sliced
- 1 tablespoon fish sauce (optional)
- 1 tablespoon lime juice
- 1 teaspoon sea salt
- 1/2 teaspoon ground black pepper
- 1/4 cup fresh cilantro, chopped

**Instructions:**

1. In a large pot, heat the olive oil over medium heat. Add the onion, garlic, and ginger, sautéing until the onion is translucent, about 5 minutes.
2. Pour in the vegetable broth and coconut milk, bringing to a simmer.
3. Add the bok choy and mushrooms, cooking for 10 minutes until tender.
4. Stir in the fish sauce (if using), lime juice, sea salt, and black pepper.
5. Simmer for another 5 minutes to combine the flavors.
6. Garnish with fresh cilantro before serving.
7. Serve hot.

**Nutrition Info (Per Serving):**

- Calories: 180
- Protein: 3g
- Carbohydrates: 10g
- Fat: 15g
- Fiber: 2g

**Serves: 4**
**Cooking Time: 25 minutes**

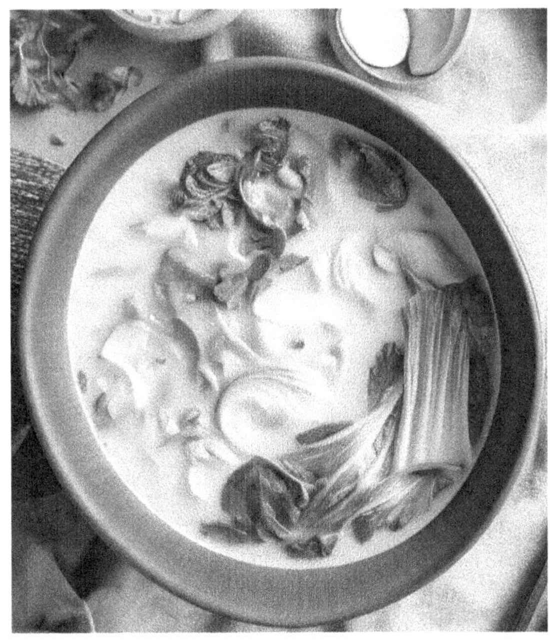

## 20. Jicama Slaw

**Ingredients:**

- 2 cups jicama, peeled and julienned
- 1 cup red cabbage, thinly sliced
- 1/2 cup carrots, julienned
- 1/4 cup red onion, thinly sliced
- 1/4 cup fresh cilantro, chopped
- 1/4 cup extra virgin olive oil
- 2 tablespoons lime juice
- 1 tablespoon honey
- 1 teaspoon ground cumin
- 1/2 teaspoon sea salt
- 1/4 teaspoon ground black pepper

**Instructions:**

1. In a large bowl, combine the jicama, red cabbage, carrots, red onion, and cilantro.
2. In a small bowl, whisk together the olive oil, lime juice, honey, ground cumin, sea salt, and black pepper.
3. Pour the dressing over the slaw, tossing to coat.
4. Serve immediately or chill for 30 minutes to let the flavors meld.

**Nutrition Info (Per Serving):**

- Calories: 120
- Protein: 1g
- Carbohydrates: 10g
- Fat: 9g
- Fiber: 4g

**Serves: 4**
**Cooking Time: 15 minutes**

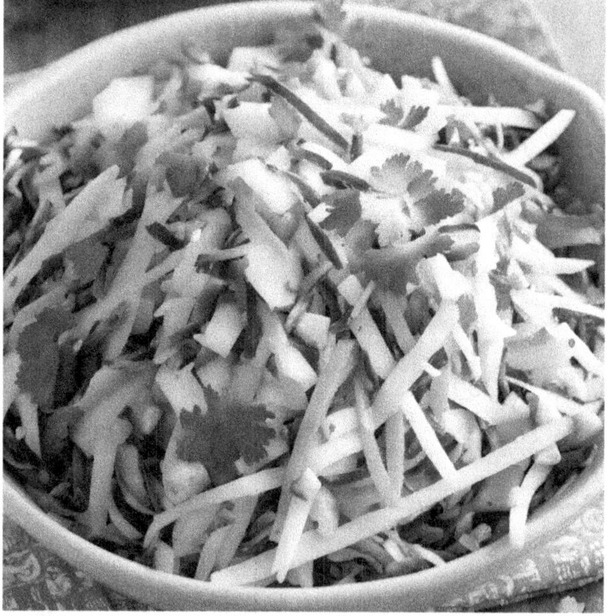

## 21. Celery Root Remoulade

**Ingredients:**

- 1 medium celery root (celeriac), peeled and julienned
- 1/2 cup coconut yogurt
- 2 tablespoons Dijon mustard
- 1 tablespoon lemon juice
- 1 tablespoon capers, drained and chopped
- 1 tablespoon fresh parsley, chopped
- 1 teaspoon apple cider vinegar
- 1/2 teaspoon sea salt
- 1/4 teaspoon ground black pepper

**Instructions:**

1. In a large bowl, combine the julienned celery root.
2. In a small bowl, whisk together the coconut yogurt, Dijon mustard, lemon juice, capers, parsley, apple cider vinegar, sea salt, and black pepper.
3. Pour the dressing over the celery root, tossing to coat.
4. Serve immediately or chill for 30 minutes to let the flavors meld.

**Nutrition Info (Per Serving):**

- Calories: 90
- Protein: 2g
- Carbohydrates: 10g
- Fat: 5g
- Fiber: 4g

**Serves: 4**
**Cooking Time: 15 minutes**

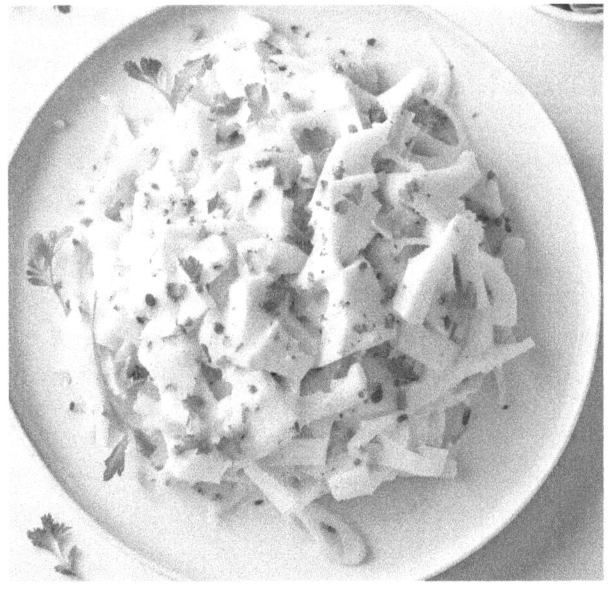

## 22. Kohlrabi Carpaccio

**Ingredients:**

- 2 medium kohlrabi, peeled and thinly sliced
- 2 tablespoons extra virgin olive oil
- 1 tablespoon lemon juice
- 1 teaspoon Dijon mustard
- 1 teaspoon honey
- 1/4 teaspoon sea salt
- 1/4 teaspoon ground black pepper
- 1/4 cup fresh parsley, chopped

**Instructions:**

1. Arrange the thinly sliced kohlrabi on a serving platter.
2. In a small bowl, whisk together the olive oil, lemon juice, Dijon mustard, honey, sea salt, and black pepper.
3. Drizzle the dressing over the kohlrabi slices.
4. Garnish with fresh parsley.
5. Serve immediately.

**Nutrition Info (Per Serving):**

- Calories: 80
- Protein: 2g
- Carbohydrates: 10g
- Fat: 4g
- Fiber: 4g

**Serves: 4**
**Cooking Time: 10 minutes**

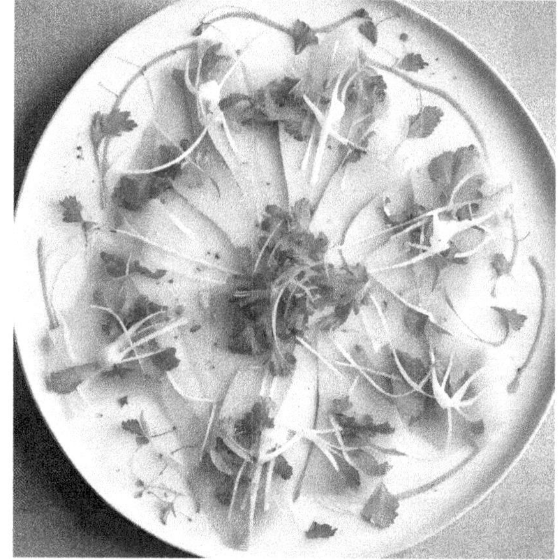

## 23. Arugula and Roasted Cauliflower Salad

**Ingredients:**

- 1 head cauliflower, cut into florets
- 3 tablespoons extra virgin olive oil, divided
- 1 teaspoon ground turmeric
- 1/2 teaspoon sea salt
- 4 cups arugula
- 1/4 cup red onion, thinly sliced
- 1/4 cup sunflower seeds, toasted
- 2 tablespoons lemon juice
- 1 teaspoon Dijon mustard
- 1/4 teaspoon ground black pepper

**Instructions:**

1. Preheat the oven to 400°F (200°C).
2. In a large bowl, toss the cauliflower florets with 1 tablespoon of olive oil, turmeric, and sea salt.
3. Spread the cauliflower on a baking sheet and roast for 25-30 minutes, until tender and golden brown.
4. In a large salad bowl, combine the arugula, roasted cauliflower, red onion, and sunflower seeds.
5. In a small bowl, whisk together the remaining olive oil, lemon juice, Dijon mustard, and black pepper.
6. Drizzle the dressing over the salad and toss to coat.
7. Serve immediately.

**Nutrition Info (Per Serving):**

- Calories: 160
- Protein: 4g
- Carbohydrates: 12g
- Fat: 12g
- Fiber: 5g

**Serves: 4**
**Cooking Time: 35 minutes**

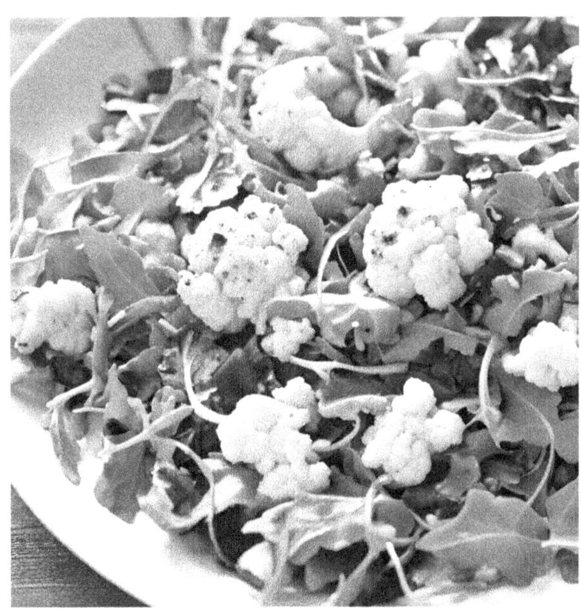

## 24. Broccoli Rabe with Olives

**Ingredients:**

- 1 bunch broccoli rabe, washed and trimmed
- 3 tablespoons extra virgin olive oil
- 2 cloves garlic, minced
- 1/4 cup Kalamata olives, pitted and sliced
- 1/2 teaspoon red pepper flakes
- 1/2 teaspoon sea salt
- 1/4 teaspoon ground black pepper

**Instructions:**

1. Bring a large pot of water to a boil. Blanch the broccoli rabe for 2-3 minutes, then drain and rinse under cold water. Set aside.
2. In a large skillet, heat the olive oil over medium heat. Add the garlic and red pepper flakes, sautéing until fragrant, about 1-2 minutes.
3. Add the blanched broccoli rabe to the skillet and sauté for 5-7 minutes, until tender.
4. Stir in the olives, sea salt, and black pepper.
5. Serve hot.

**Nutrition Info (Per Serving):**

- Calories: 150
- Protein: 4g
- Carbohydrates: 8g
- Fat: 12g
- Fiber: 4g

**Serves: 4**
**Cooking Time: 15 minutes**

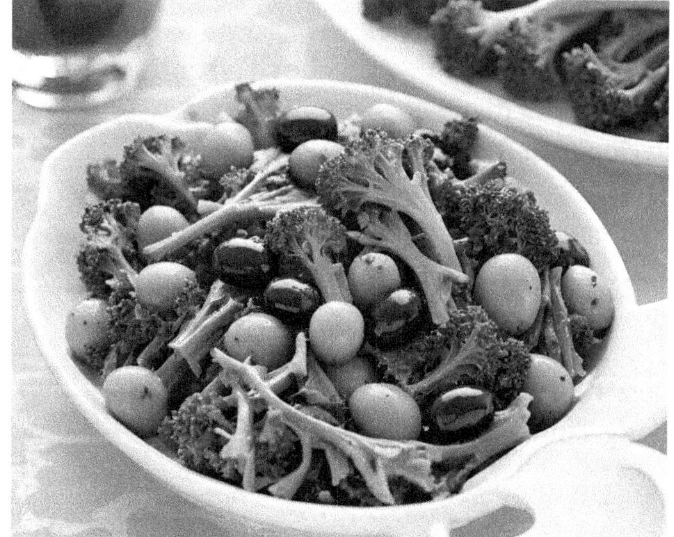

## 25. Creamy Avocado and Spinach Dip

**Ingredients:**

- 2 ripe avocados
- 2 cups fresh spinach, washed
- 2 cloves garlic, minced
- 2 tablespoons lemon juice
- 1 tablespoon extra virgin olive oil
- 1/2 teaspoon sea salt
- 1/4 teaspoon ground black pepper

**Instructions:**

1. In a food processor, combine the avocados, spinach, garlic, lemon juice, and olive oil.
2. Blend until smooth and creamy.
3. Season with sea salt and black pepper.
4. Serve immediately with fresh vegetable sticks or lectin-free crackers.

**Nutrition Info (Per Serving):**

- Calories: 180
- Protein: 2g
- Carbohydrates: 10g
- Fat: 15g
- Fiber: 7g

**Serves: 4**

**Cooking Time: 10 minutes**

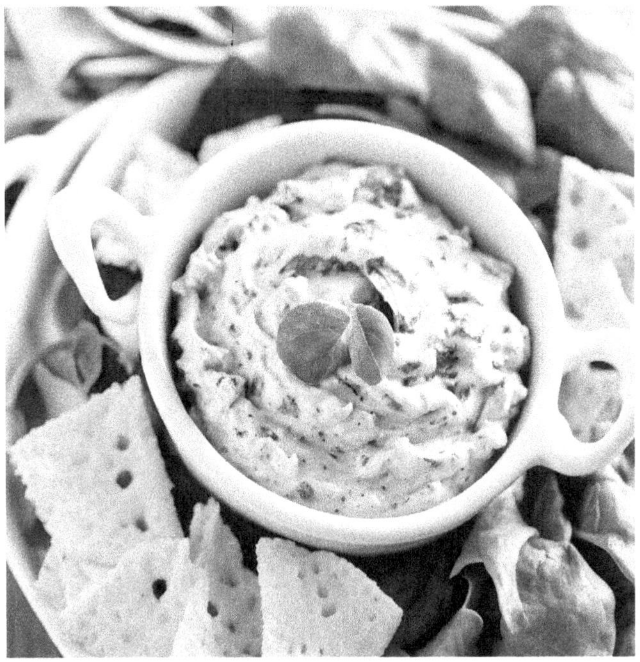

## 26. Carrot and Cucumber Nori Rolls

**Ingredients:**

- 4 nori sheets
- 1 large carrot, julienned
- 1 large cucumber, julienned
- 1 avocado, sliced
- 1/4 cup fresh cilantro, chopped
- 1 tablespoon sesame seeds
- 1 tablespoon coconut aminos

**Instructions:**

1. Lay out a nori sheet on a flat surface.
2. Arrange a small amount of carrot, cucumber, avocado, and cilantro on the nori sheet, about 1 inch from the bottom edge.
3. Sprinkle with sesame seeds.
4. Carefully roll the nori sheet from the bottom, keeping the filling tight.
5. Slice each roll into 4 pieces.
6. Serve with coconut aminos for dipping.

**Nutrition Info (Per Serving):**

- Calories: 70
- Protein: 2g
- Carbohydrates: 10g
- Fat: 4g
- Fiber: 3g

**Serves: 4**
**Cooking Time: 15 minutes**

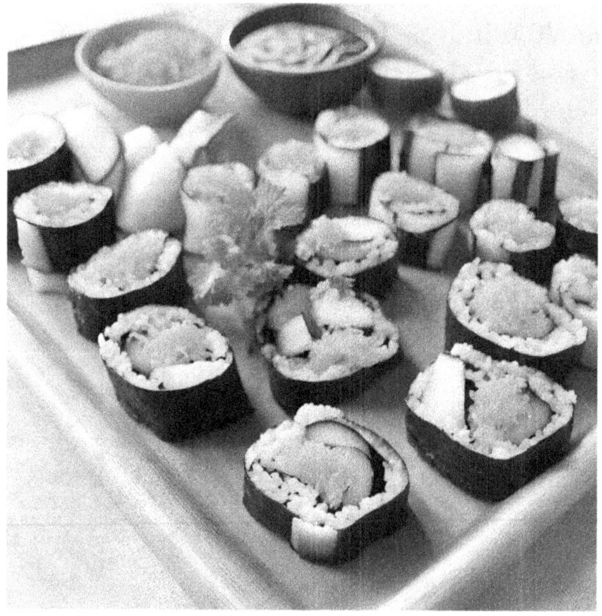

## 27. Turnip and Apple Purée

**Ingredients:**

- 4 medium turnips, peeled and chopped
- 2 large apples, peeled, cored, and chopped
- 1/4 cup coconut milk
- 2 tablespoons extra virgin olive oil
- 1/2 teaspoon ground cinnamon
- 1/2 teaspoon sea salt
- 1/4 teaspoon ground black pepper

**Instructions:**

1. In a large pot, combine the turnips and apples. Add enough water to cover and bring to a boil.
2. Reduce heat and simmer until tender, about 15-20 minutes. Drain.
3. Transfer the turnips and apples to a food processor. Add the coconut milk, olive oil, cinnamon, sea salt, and black pepper.
4. Blend until smooth and creamy.
5. Serve warm.

**Nutrition Info (Per Serving):**

- Calories: 120
- Protein: 1g
- Carbohydrates: 15g
- Fat: 7g
- Fiber: 3g

**Serves: 4**
**Cooking Time: 25 minutes**

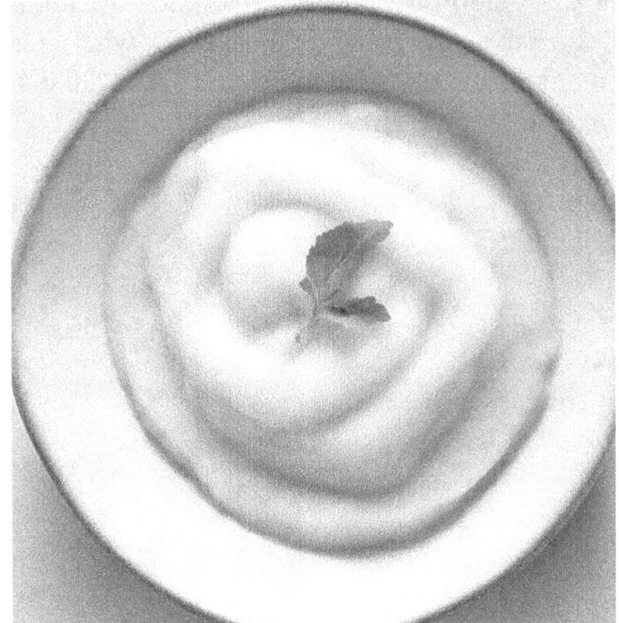

# Fish and Seafood Recipes

**1. Grilled Salmon with Dill**

**Ingredients**:

- 4 salmon fillets (about 6 ounces each)
- 2 tablespoons extra virgin olive oil
- 2 tablespoons fresh dill, chopped
- 1 tablespoon lemon juice
- 2 cloves garlic, minced
- 1 teaspoon sea salt
- 1/2 teaspoon ground black pepper

**Instructions:**

1. Preheat the grill to medium-high heat.
2. In a small bowl, mix the olive oil, dill, lemon juice, garlic, sea salt, and black pepper.
3. Brush the mixture over both sides of the salmon fillets.
4. Place the salmon on the grill and cook for about 4-5 minutes on each side, or until the fish is opaque and flakes easily with a fork.
5. Serve hot, garnished with additional fresh dill if desired.

**Nutrition Info (Per Serving):**

- Calories: 320
- Protein: 34g
- Carbohydrates: 1g
- Fat: 20g
- Fiber: 0g

**Serves: 4**

**Cooking Time: 15 minutes**

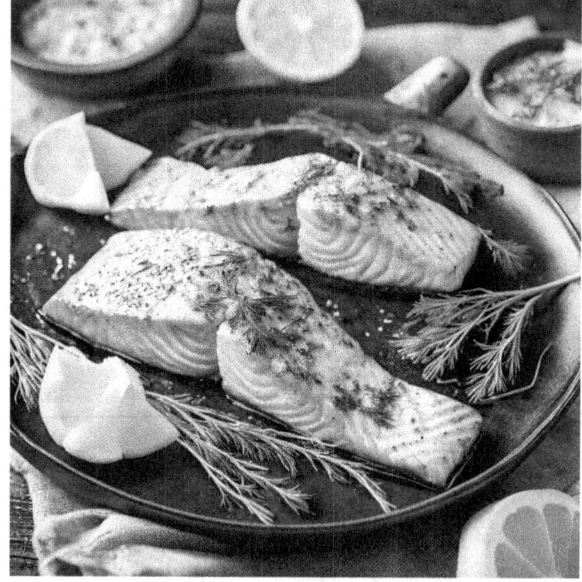

## 2. Baked Cod with Lemon and Herbs

**Ingredients:**

- 4 cod fillets (about 6 ounces each)
- 3 tablespoons extra virgin olive oil
- 2 tablespoons fresh parsley, chopped
- 1 tablespoon fresh thyme, chopped
- 1 tablespoon lemon zest
- 2 cloves garlic, minced
- 1 teaspoon sea salt
- 1/2 teaspoon ground black pepper

**Instructions:**

1. Preheat the oven to 375°F (190°C).
2. In a small bowl, mix the olive oil, parsley, thyme, lemon zest, garlic, sea salt, and black pepper.
3. Place the cod fillets in a baking dish and brush the herb mixture evenly over each fillet.
4. Bake for 15-20 minutes, or until the fish is opaque and flakes easily with a fork.
5. Serve hot, garnished with lemon slices if desired.

**Nutrition Info (Per Serving):**

- Calories: 220
- Protein: 32g
- Carbohydrates: 1g
- Fat: 10g
- Fiber: 0g

**Serves: 4**
**Cooking Time: 20 minutes**

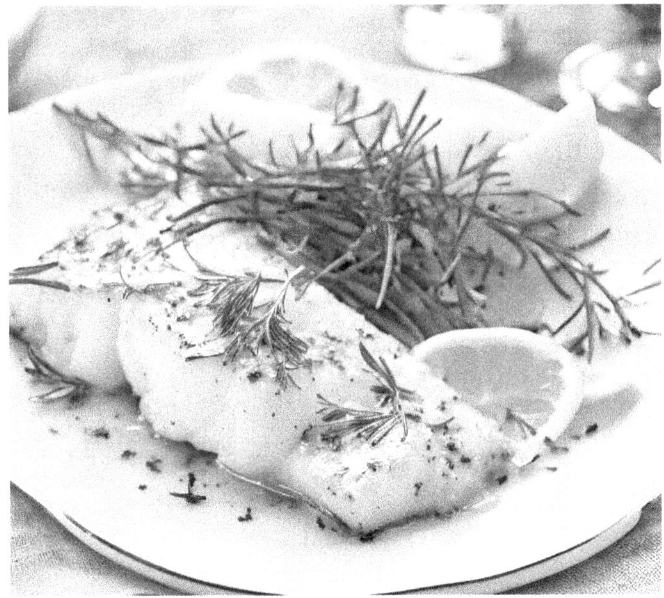

## 3. Oven-Roasted Trout with Thyme

**Ingredients:**

- 4 whole trout, cleaned and gutted
- 4 tablespoons extra virgin olive oil
- 4 sprigs fresh thyme
- 2 lemons, thinly sliced
- 4 cloves garlic, minced
- 1 teaspoon sea salt
- 1/2 teaspoon ground black pepper

**Instructions:**

1. Preheat the oven to 400°F (200°C).
2. Place the trout on a baking sheet lined with parchment paper.
3. Drizzle 1 tablespoon of olive oil inside each trout. Place a sprig of thyme and a few lemon slices inside each fish.
4. In a small bowl, mix the minced garlic, sea salt, and black pepper. Rub this mixture over the outside of each trout.
5. Arrange the remaining lemon slices around the fish.
6. Roast in the preheated oven for 20-25 minutes, or until the fish is opaque and flakes easily with a fork.
7. Serve hot, garnished with additional thyme if desired.

**Nutrition Info (Per Serving):**

- Calories: 310
- Protein: 34g
- Carbohydrates: 2g
- Fat: 18g
- Fiber: 1g

**Serves: 4**

**Cooking Time: 30 minutes**

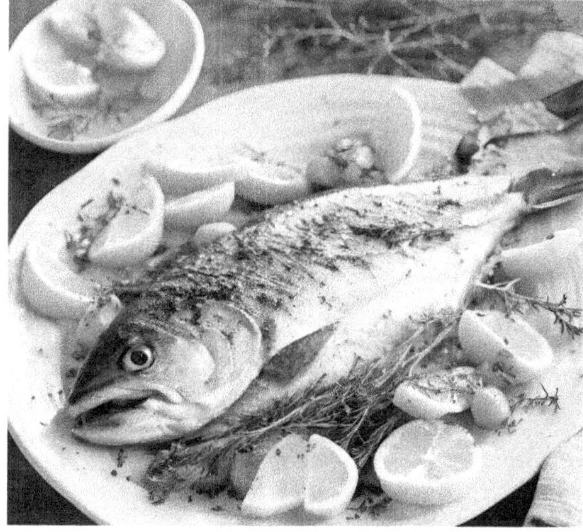

## 4. Grilled Tuna Steaks with Olive Oil

**Ingredients:**

- 4 tuna steaks (about 6 ounces each)
- 3 tablespoons extra virgin olive oil
- 2 tablespoons fresh basil, chopped
- 1 tablespoon lemon juice
- 2 cloves garlic, minced
- 1 teaspoon sea salt
- 1/2 teaspoon ground black pepper

**Instructions:**

1. Preheat the grill to high heat.
2. In a small bowl, mix the olive oil, basil, lemon juice, garlic, sea salt, and black pepper.
3. Brush the mixture over both sides of the tuna steaks.
4. Place the tuna steaks on the grill and cook for about 3-4 minutes on each side, or until the desired doneness is reached.
5. Serve hot, garnished with additional fresh basil if desired.

**Nutrition Info (Per Serving):**

- Calories: 280
- Protein: 37g
- Carbohydrates: 1g
- Fat: 14g
- Fiber: 0g

**Serves: 4**
**Cooking Time: 10 minutes**

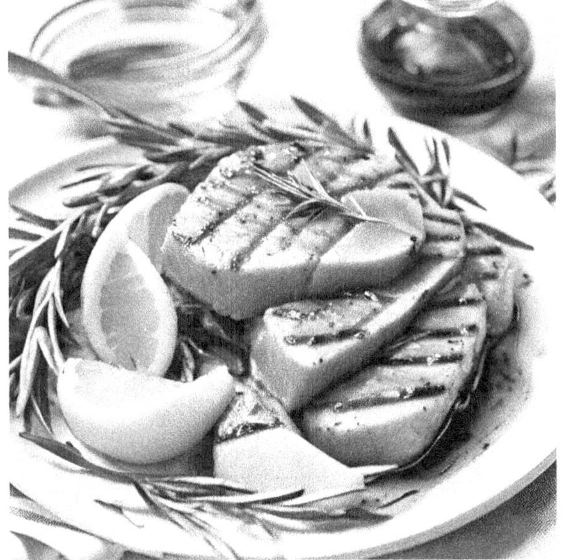

## 5. Fisherman's Stew with Halibut

**Ingredients:**

- 1 lb halibut fillets, cut into chunks
- 2 tablespoons extra virgin olive oil
- 1 large onion, chopped
- 3 cloves garlic, minced
- 2 cups vegetable broth
- 1 cup water
- 1 cup chopped celery
- 1 cup chopped carrots
- 1 cup chopped fennel
- 1/4 cup fresh parsley, chopped
- 1 tablespoon fresh thyme, chopped
- 1/2 teaspoon sea salt
- 1/4 teaspoon ground black pepper

**Instructions:**

1. In a large pot, heat the olive oil over medium heat. Add the onion and garlic, sautéing until translucent, about 5 minutes.
2. Add the vegetable broth, water, celery, carrots, and fennel. Bring to a boil, then reduce heat and simmer for 15 minutes.
3. Add the halibut chunks, parsley, thyme, sea salt, and black pepper. Simmer for another 10-12 minutes, until the fish is cooked through and flakes easily with a fork.
4. Serve hot.

**Nutrition Info (Per Serving):**

- Calories: 220
- Protein: 25g
- Carbohydrates: 12g
- Fat: 8g
- Fiber: 3g

**Serves: 4**

**Cooking Time: 35 minutes**

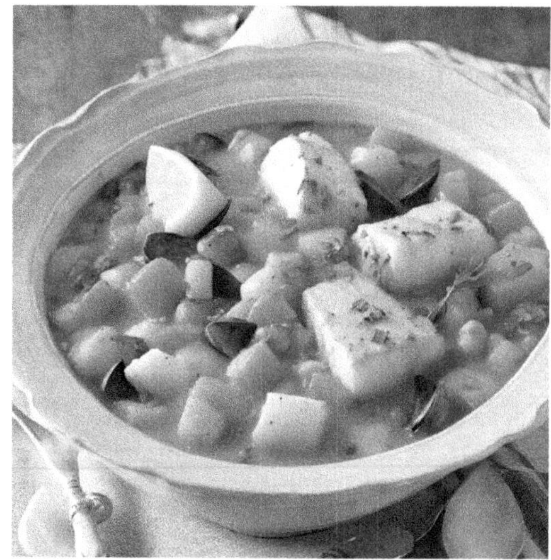

## 6. Clam Soup with Garlic and Herbs

**Ingredients:**

- 2 lbs fresh clams, scrubbed
- 2 tablespoons extra virgin olive oil
- 1 large onion, finely chopped
- 4 cloves garlic, minced
- 4 cups low-sodium chicken broth
- 1 cup water
- 1/4 cup fresh parsley, chopped
- 2 tablespoons fresh dill, chopped
- 1 teaspoon sea salt
- 1/2 teaspoon ground black pepper

**Instructions:**

1. In a large pot, heat the olive oil over medium heat. Add the onion and garlic, sautéing until translucent, about 5 minutes.
2. Add the chicken broth and water, bringing to a boil.
3. Add the clams, cover, and cook for 5-7 minutes, until the clams open. Discard any that do not open.
4. Stir in the parsley, dill, sea salt, and black pepper.
5. Serve hot.

**Nutrition Info (Per Serving):**

- Calories: 180
- Protein: 24g
- Carbohydrates: 6g
- Fat: 6g
- Fiber: 1g

**Serves: 4**
**Cooking Time: 20 minutes**

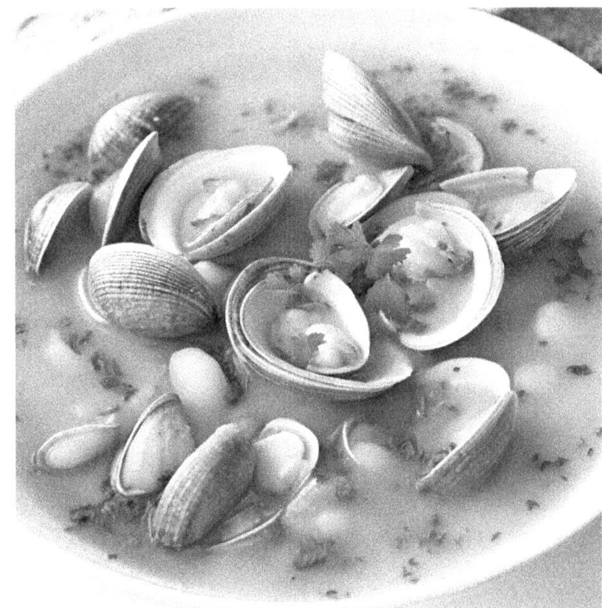

## 7. Shrimp Broth with Fennel

**Ingredients:**

- 1 lb shrimp, peeled and deveined
- 2 tablespoons extra virgin olive oil
- 1 large fennel bulb, thinly sliced
- 1 large onion, chopped
- 3 cloves garlic, minced
- 4 cups low-sodium chicken broth
- 1 cup water
- 1 tablespoon lemon juice
- 1/4 cup fresh parsley, chopped
- 1 teaspoon sea salt
- 1/2 teaspoon ground black pepper

Instructions:

1. In a large pot, heat the olive oil over medium heat. Add the fennel, onion, and garlic, sautéing until translucent, about 5 minutes.
2. Add the chicken broth and water, bringing to a boil.
3. Add the shrimp and lemon juice, simmering for 5-7 minutes until the shrimp is pink and cooked through.
4. Stir in the parsley, sea salt, and black pepper.
5. Serve hot.

**Nutrition Info (Per Serving):**

- Calories: 180
- Protein: 22g
- Carbohydrates: 6g
- Fat: 8g
- Fiber: 1g

**Serves: 4**

**Cooking Time: 20 minutes**

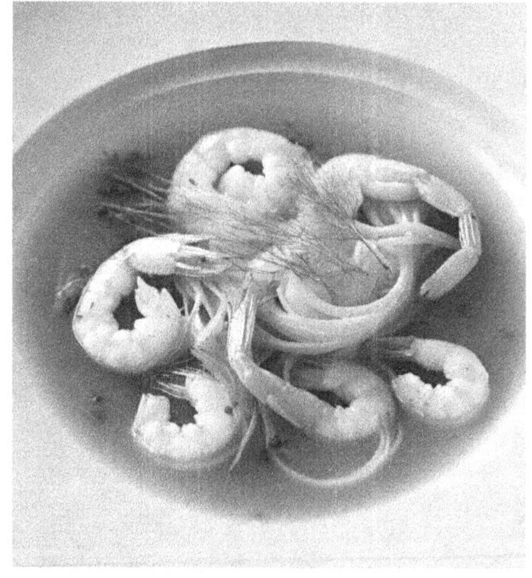

## 8. Shrimp Sautéed with Spinach

**Ingredients:**

- 1 lb shrimp, peeled and deveined
- 3 tablespoons extra virgin olive oil
- 3 cloves garlic, minced
- 1 large onion, finely chopped
- 6 cups fresh spinach, washed
- 1 tablespoon lemon juice
- 1 teaspoon sea salt
- 1/2 teaspoon ground black pepper

**Instructions:**

1. In a large skillet, heat the olive oil over medium heat. Add the garlic and onion, sautéing until translucent, about 5 minutes.
2. Add the shrimp and cook for 3-4 minutes, until pink and opaque.
3. Add the spinach, lemon juice, sea salt, and black pepper, cooking for another 2-3 minutes until the spinach is wilted.
4. Serve hot.

**Nutrition Info (Per Serving):**

- Calories: 220
- Protein: 24g
- Carbohydrates: 6g
- Fat: 12g
- Fiber: 3g

**Serves: 4**
**Cooking Time: 15 minutes**

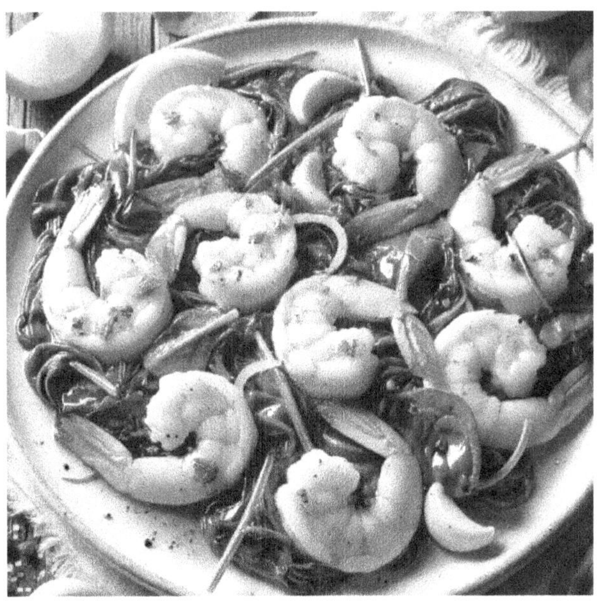

## 9. Sardines Fried in Olive Oil

**Ingredients:**

- 1 lb fresh sardines, cleaned and gutted
- 1/4 cup extra virgin olive oil
- 1/4 cup fresh parsley, chopped
- 2 cloves garlic, minced
- 1 tablespoon lemon juice
- 1 teaspoon sea salt
- 1/2 teaspoon ground black pepper

**Instructions:**

1. In a large skillet, heat the olive oil over medium heat.
2. Add the garlic and cook for 1-2 minutes until fragrant.
3. Add the sardines and cook for 3-4 minutes on each side, until crispy and golden brown.
4. Remove from heat and sprinkle with parsley, lemon juice, sea salt, and black pepper.
5. Serve hot.

**Nutrition Info (Per Serving):**

- Calories: 250
- Protein: 25g
- Carbohydrates: 1g
- Fat: 16g
- Fiber: 0g

**Serves: 4**

**Cooking Time: 15 minutes**

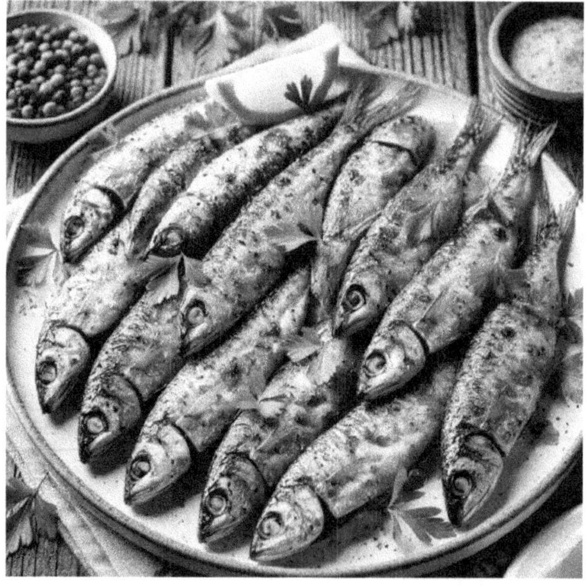

## 10. Crab Stir-Fry with Ginger

**Ingredients:**

- 1 lb fresh crab meat
- 3 tablespoons extra virgin olive oil
- 1 large onion, chopped
- 2 cloves garlic, minced
- 1 tablespoon fresh ginger, grated
- 1 cup snap peas, trimmed
- 1 red bell pepper, thinly sliced
- 2 tablespoons coconut aminos
- 1 teaspoon sea salt
- 1/2 teaspoon ground black pepper
- 1/4 cup fresh cilantro, chopped

**Instructions:**

1. In a large skillet, heat the olive oil over medium heat. Add the onion, garlic, and ginger, sautéing until fragrant, about 3-4 minutes.
2. Add the snap peas and bell pepper, cooking for 5-7 minutes until tender.
3. Stir in the crab meat, coconut aminos, sea salt, and black pepper. Cook for another 3-4 minutes until heated through.
4. Garnish with fresh cilantro before serving.
5. Serve hot.

**Nutrition Info (Per Serving):**

- Calories: 220
- Protein: 20g
- Carbohydrates: 8g
- Fat: 12g
- Fiber: 2g

**Serves: 4**
**Cooking Time: 20 minutes**

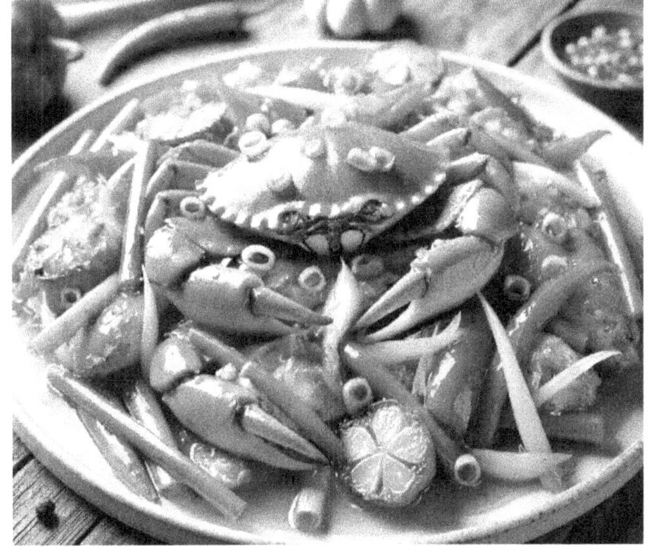

**11. Ceviche with Snapper and Lime**

**Ingredients:**

- 1 lb snapper fillets, cut into small cubes
- 1/2 cup fresh lime juice
- 1/4 cup fresh lemon juice
- 1/4 cup red onion, finely chopped
- 1/4 cup fresh cilantro, chopped
- 1 jalapeño pepper, seeded and minced (optional)
- 1 cucumber, peeled, seeded, and diced
- 1 avocado, diced
- 1 teaspoon sea salt
- 1/4 teaspoon ground black pepper

**Instructions:**

1. In a glass bowl, combine the snapper cubes, lime juice, and lemon juice. Ensure the fish is fully submerged. Cover and refrigerate for 1-2 hours, until the fish turns opaque.
2. Drain the fish, discarding most of the marinade but leaving a little for flavor.
3. Add the red onion, cilantro, jalapeño (if using), cucumber, avocado, sea salt, and black pepper. Toss gently to combine.
4. Serve immediately.

**Nutrition Info (Per Serving):**

- Calories: 180
- Protein: 20g
- Carbohydrates: 10g
- Fat: 7g
- Fiber: 4g

**Serves: 4**

**Cooking Time: 2 hours (including marinating time)**

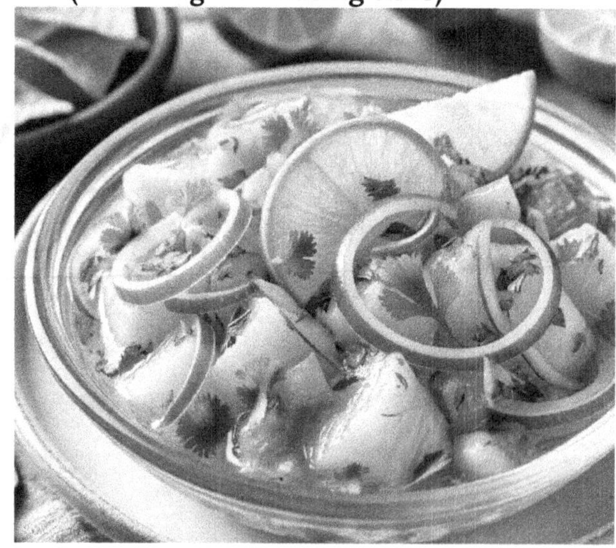

## 12. Tuna Tartare with Avocado

**Ingredients:**

- 1 lb sushi-grade tuna, diced
- 1 avocado, diced
- 2 tablespoons extra virgin olive oil
- 1 tablespoon fresh lime juice
- 1 tablespoon coconut aminos
- 1 teaspoon fresh ginger, grated
- 1 teaspoon sesame oil
- 1/4 cup green onions, finely chopped
- 1/4 cup fresh cilantro, chopped
- 1 teaspoon sea salt
- 1/4 teaspoon ground black pepper

**Instructions:**

1. In a large bowl, combine the tuna, avocado, olive oil, lime juice, coconut aminos, ginger, sesame oil, green onions, cilantro, sea salt, and black pepper.
2. Gently toss to combine all ingredients.
3. Serve immediately, either on its own or with lettuce leaves for wrapping.

**Nutrition Info (Per Serving):**

- Calories: 250
- Protein: 25g
- Carbohydrates: 7g
- Fat: 15g
- Fiber: 3g

**Serves: 4**
**Cooking Time: 10 minutes**

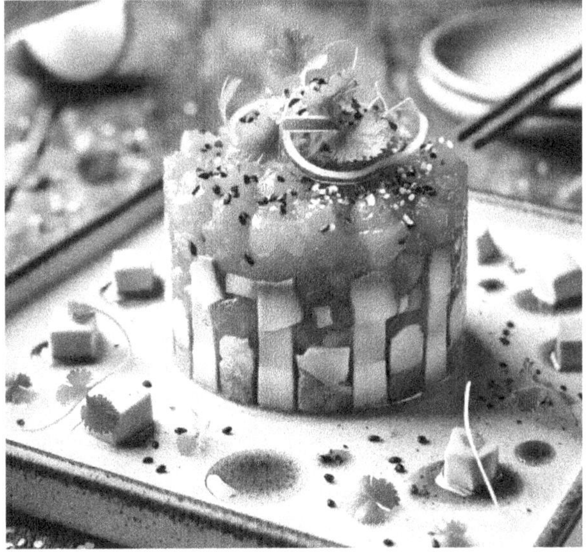

## 13. Oysters with a Vinegar Mignonette

**Ingredients:**

- 12 fresh oysters, shucked
- 1/4 cup red wine vinegar
- 2 tablespoons shallots, finely minced
- 1 tablespoon fresh parsley, chopped
- 1 teaspoon black peppercorns, crushed
- 1/4 teaspoon sea salt

**Instructions:**

1. In a small bowl, combine the red wine vinegar, shallots, parsley, crushed black peppercorns, and sea salt. Mix well.
2. Arrange the shucked oysters on a platter.
3. Spoon a small amount of the mignonette sauce over each oyster.
4. Serve immediately.

**Nutrition Info (Per Serving):**

- Calories: 50
- Protein: 5g
- Carbohydrates: 2g
- Fat: 1g
- Fiber: 0g

**Serves: 4**
**Cooking Time: 10 minutes**

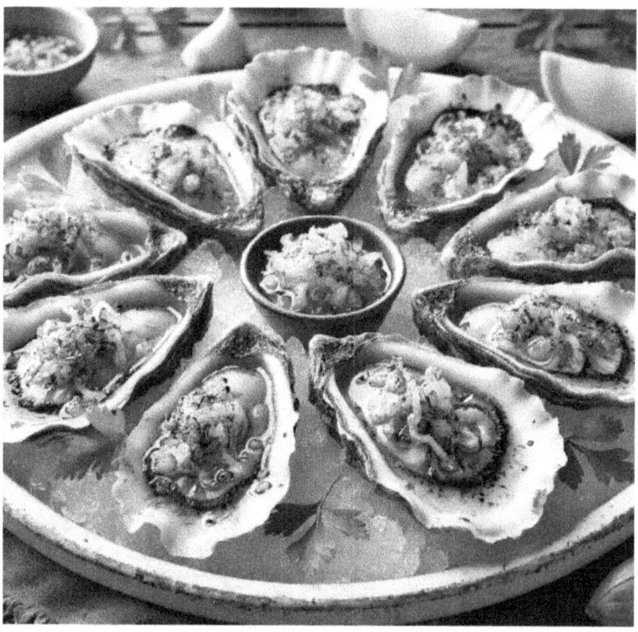

## 14. Barbecue Shrimp Skewers

**Ingredients:**

- 1 lb large shrimp, peeled and deveined
- 2 tablespoons extra virgin olive oil
- 2 tablespoons fresh lemon juice
- 2 cloves garlic, minced
- 1 tablespoon fresh parsley, chopped
- 1 teaspoon paprika
- 1/2 teaspoon sea salt
- 1/4 teaspoon ground black pepper
- Wooden skewers, soaked in water for 30 minutes

**Instructions:**

1. Preheat the grill to medium-high heat.
2. In a large bowl, combine the olive oil, lemon juice, garlic, parsley, paprika, sea salt, and black pepper. Mix well.
3. Add the shrimp to the bowl and toss to coat evenly with the marinade. Let sit for 10 minutes.
4. Thread the shrimp onto the soaked wooden skewers.
5. Grill the shrimp skewers for 2-3 minutes on each side, until the shrimp are pink and opaque.
6. Serve hot.

**Nutrition Info (Per Serving):**

- Calories: 180
- Protein: 24g
- Carbohydrates: 2g
- Fat: 8g
- Fiber: 0g

**Serves: 4**
**Cooking Time: 15 minutes**

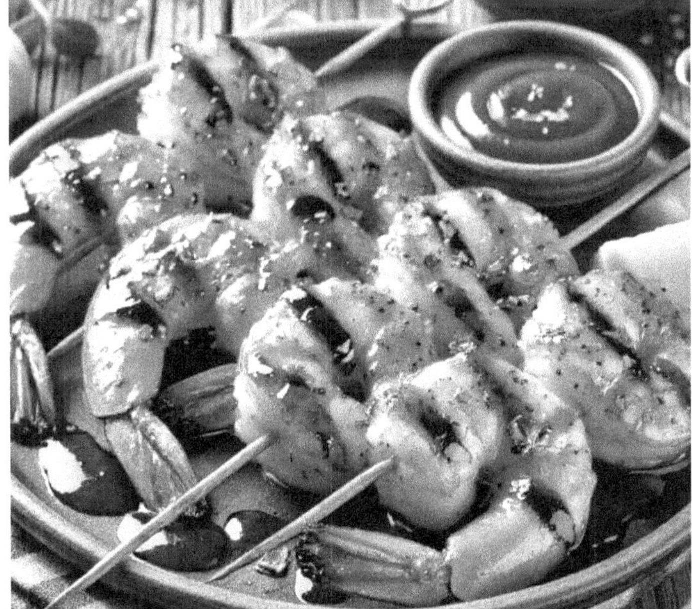

## 15. Char-Grilled Octopus with Olive Oil

**Ingredients:**

- 2 pounds octopus, cleaned
- 1/4 cup extra virgin olive oil
- 2 cloves garlic, minced
- 1 tablespoon fresh lemon juice
- 1 teaspoon fresh thyme, chopped
- 1 teaspoon sea salt
- 1/2 teaspoon ground black pepper
- 1/4 cup fresh parsley, chopped

**Instructions:**

1. Bring a large pot of water to a boil. Add the cleaned octopus and cook for 45-60 minutes, until tender. Drain and let cool.
2. Preheat the grill to high heat.
3. In a small bowl, mix the olive oil, garlic, lemon juice, thyme, sea salt, and black pepper.
4. Brush the octopus with the olive oil mixture.
5. Grill the octopus for 3-4 minutes on each side, until charred and crispy.
6. Remove from the grill and sprinkle with fresh parsley.
7. Serve hot.

**Nutrition Info (Per Serving):**

- Calories: 220
- Protein: 28g
- Carbohydrates: 2g
- Fat: 11g
- Fiber: 0g

**Serves: 4**

**Cooking Time: 1 hour 20 minutes (including boiling time)**

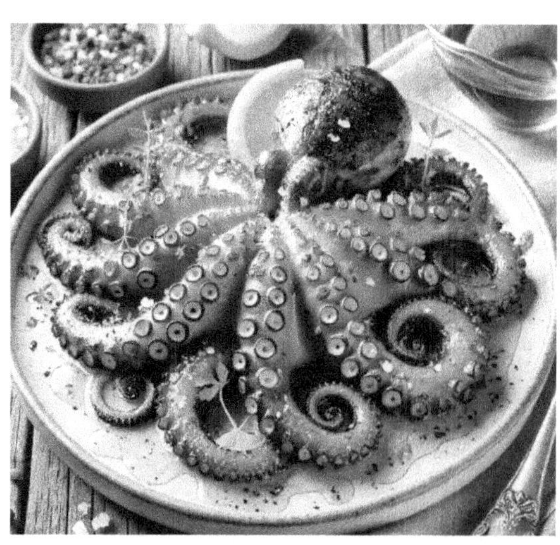

## 16. Grilled Mahi-Mahi with Lime

**Ingredients:**

- 4 mahi-mahi fillets (about 6 ounces each)
- 3 tablespoons extra virgin olive oil
- 2 tablespoons fresh lime juice
- 2 cloves garlic, minced
- 1 tablespoon fresh cilantro, chopped
- 1 teaspoon sea salt
- 1/2 teaspoon ground black pepper

**Instructions:**

1. Preheat the grill to medium-high heat.
2. In a small bowl, mix the olive oil, lime juice, garlic, cilantro, sea salt, and black pepper.
3. Brush the mixture over both sides of the mahi-mahi fillets.
4. Grill the mahi-mahi for about 4-5 minutes on each side, or until the fish is opaque and flakes easily with a fork.
5. Serve hot, garnished with additional fresh cilantro if desired.

**Nutrition Info (Per Serving):**

- Calories: 240
- Protein: 36g
- Carbohydrates: 2g
- Fat: 10g
- Fiber: 0g

**Serves: 4**

**Cooking Time: 15 minutes**

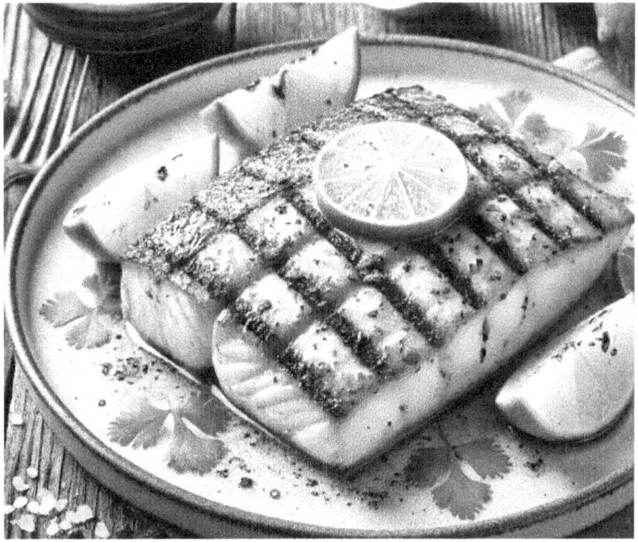

## 17. Shrimp Salad with Mixed Greens

**Ingredients:**

- 1 lb shrimp, peeled and deveined
- 3 tablespoons extra virgin olive oil
- 1 tablespoon fresh lemon juice
- 1 teaspoon Dijon mustard
- 4 cups mixed greens (arugula, spinach, kale)
- 1/2 cup red onion, thinly sliced
- 1 avocado, sliced
- 1/4 cup fresh parsley, chopped
- 1 teaspoon sea salt
- 1/2 teaspoon ground black pepper

**Instructions:**

1. In a large skillet, heat 1 tablespoon of olive oil over medium heat. Add the shrimp and cook for 3-4 minutes, until pink and opaque. Remove from heat and let cool.
2. In a small bowl, whisk together the remaining olive oil, lemon juice, Dijon mustard, sea salt, and black pepper.
3. In a large salad bowl, combine the mixed greens, red onion, avocado, and parsley. Add the cooked shrimp.
4. Drizzle the dressing over the salad and toss gently to combine.
5. Serve immediately.

**Nutrition Info (Per Serving):**

- Calories: 280
- Protein: 24g
- Carbohydrates: 10g
- Fat: 18g
- Fiber: 6g

**Serves: 4**

**Cooking Time: 15 minutes**

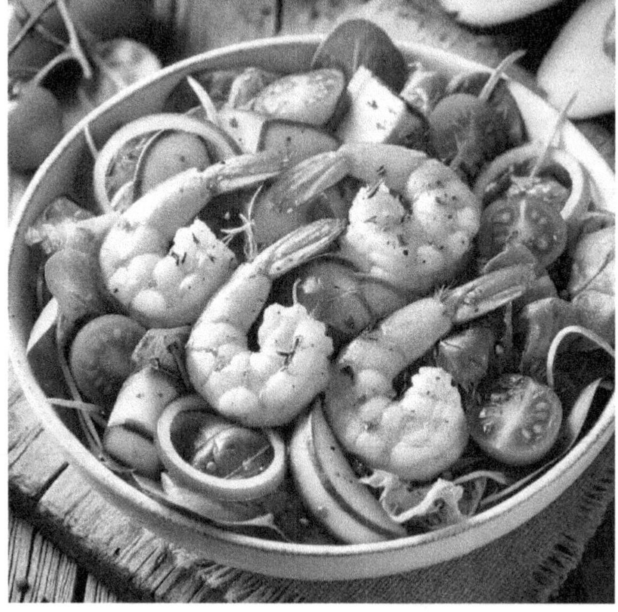

## 18. Crab Salad with Celery

**Ingredients:**

- 1 lb fresh crab meat
- 1/2 cup celery, finely chopped
- 1/4 cup red onion, finely chopped
- 1/4 cup mayonnaise (made with avocado oil)
- 2 tablespoons fresh lemon juice
- 1 tablespoon fresh dill, chopped
- 1 teaspoon Dijon mustard
- 1 teaspoon sea salt
- 1/2 teaspoon ground black pepper

**Instructions:**

1. In a large bowl, combine the crab meat, celery, and red onion.
2. In a small bowl, whisk together the mayonnaise, lemon juice, dill, Dijon mustard, sea salt, and black pepper.
3. Pour the dressing over the crab mixture and gently toss to combine.
4. Serve immediately or chill for 30 minutes to let the flavors meld.

**Nutrition Info (Per Serving):**

- Calories: 200
- Protein: 22g
- Carbohydrates: 3g
- Fat: 12g
- Fiber: 1g

**Serves: 4**
**Cooking Time: 10 minute**

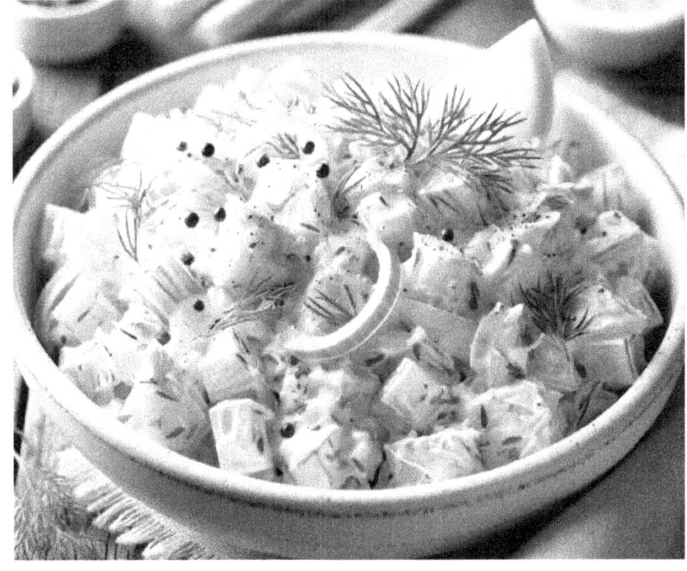

## 19. Smoked Salmon Salad with Arugula

**Ingredients:**

- 8 ounces smoked salmon, sliced
- 4 cups arugula
- 1/2 cup red onion, thinly sliced
- 1/4 cup capers, drained
- 1 avocado, sliced
- 3 tablespoons extra virgin olive oil
- 1 tablespoon fresh lemon juice
- 1 teaspoon Dijon mustard
- 1/4 teaspoon sea salt
- 1/4 teaspoon ground black pepper

**Instructions:**

1. In a large salad bowl, combine the arugula, red onion, capers, and avocado.
2. In a small bowl, whisk together the olive oil, lemon juice, Dijon mustard, sea salt, and black pepper.
3. Drizzle the dressing over the salad and toss gently to combine.
4. Top the salad with the smoked salmon slices.
5. Serve immediately.

**Nutrition Info (Per Serving):**

- Calories: 250
- Protein: 14g
- Carbohydrates: 8g
- Fat: 18g
- Fiber: 4g

**Serves: 4**

**Cooking Time: 10 minutes**

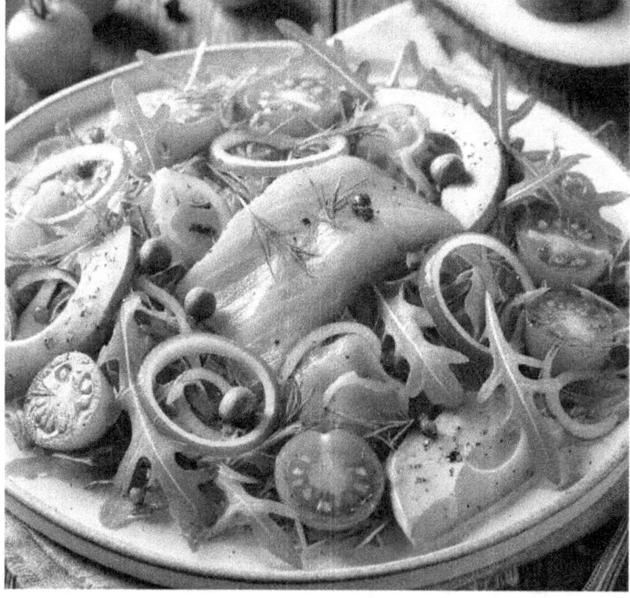

## 20. Indian Fish Curry with Coconut Milk

**Ingredients:**

- 1 lb white fish fillets (such as cod or tilapia), cut into chunks
- 2 tablespoons extra virgin olive oil
- 1 large onion, finely chopped
- 3 cloves garlic, minced
- 1 tablespoon fresh ginger, grated
- 1 tablespoon curry powder
- 1 teaspoon ground turmeric
- 1 teaspoon ground cumin
- 1 teaspoon ground coriander
- 1 can (14 oz) coconut milk
- 1/2 cup vegetable broth
- 1 tablespoon fresh lemon juice
- 1/4 cup fresh cilantro, chopped
- 1 teaspoon sea salt
- 1/4 teaspoon ground black pepper

**Instructions:**

1. In a large skillet, heat the olive oil over medium heat. Add the onion, garlic, and ginger, sautéing until the onion is translucent, about 5 minutes.
2. Add the curry powder, turmeric, cumin, and coriander, cooking for another 2 minutes until fragrant.
3. Pour in the coconut milk and vegetable broth, bringing to a simmer.
4. Add the fish chunks, lemon juice, sea salt, and black pepper. Simmer for 10-12 minutes, until the fish is cooked through and flakes easily.
5. Stir in the fresh cilantro.
6. Serve hot.

**Nutrition Info (Per Serving):**

- Calories: 320
- Protein: 25g
- Carbohydrates: 8g
- Fat: 22g
- Fiber: 2g

**Serves: 4**

**Cooking Time: 30 minutes**

## 21. Greek Style Grilled Octopus

**Ingredients:**

- 2 pounds octopus, cleaned
- 1/4 cup extra virgin olive oil
- 2 tablespoons fresh lemon juice
- 2 cloves garlic, minced
- 1 tablespoon fresh oregano, chopped
- 1 teaspoon sea salt
- 1/2 teaspoon ground black pepper
- 1/4 cup fresh parsley, chopped

**Instructions:**

1. Bring a large pot of water to a boil. Add the cleaned octopus and cook for 45-60 minutes, until tender. Drain and let cool.
2. Preheat the grill to high heat.
3. In a small bowl, mix the olive oil, lemon juice, garlic, oregano, sea salt, and black pepper.
4. Brush the octopus with the olive oil mixture.
5. Grill the octopus for 3-4 minutes on each side, until charred and crispy.
6. Remove from the grill and sprinkle with fresh parsley.
7. Serve hot.

**Nutrition Info (Per Serving):**

- Calories: 250
- Protein: 30g
- Carbohydrates: 3g
- Fat: 12g
- Fiber: 1g

**Serves: 4**

**Cooking Time: 1 hour 20 minutes (including boiling time)**

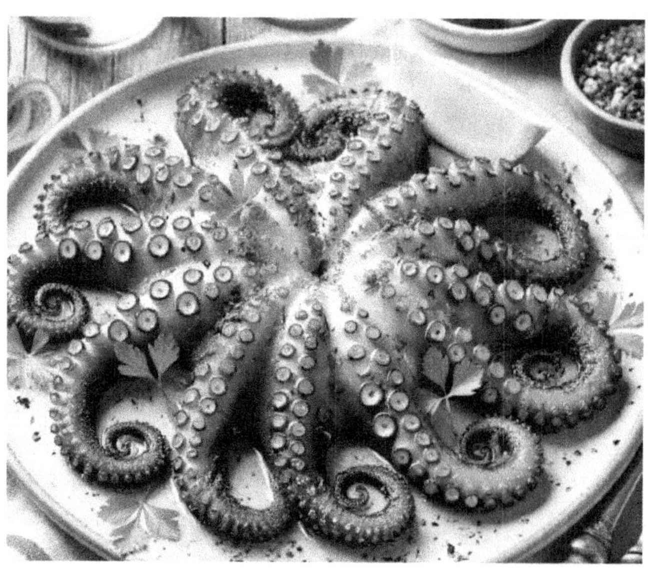

## 22. Japanese Seaweed and Seafood Salad

**Ingredients:**

- 1 cup dried seaweed (wakame), soaked and drained
- 1/2 lb shrimp, peeled and deveined
- 1/2 lb scallops
- 1/4 cup extra virgin olive oil
- 2 tablespoons rice vinegar
- 1 tablespoon tamari (gluten-free soy sauce)
- 1 teaspoon sesame oil
- 1 tablespoon fresh ginger, grated
- 1 clove garlic, minced
- 1 teaspoon sea salt
- 1/4 teaspoon ground black pepper
- 1/4 cup green onions, chopped
- 1 tablespoon sesame seeds

**Instructions:**

1. Bring a large pot of water to a boil. Add the shrimp and scallops, cooking for 3-4 minutes until opaque. Drain and let cool.
2. In a large bowl, combine the soaked seaweed, shrimp, and scallops.
3. In a small bowl, whisk together the olive oil, rice vinegar, tamari, sesame oil, ginger, garlic, sea salt, and black pepper.
4. Pour the dressing over the seaweed and seafood mixture, tossing to coat.
5. Garnish with green onions and sesame seeds.
6. Serve chilled.

**Nutrition Info (Per Serving):**

- Calories: 200
- Protein: 20g
- Carbohydrates: 6g
- Fat: 12g
- Fiber: 3g

**Serves: 4**

**Cooking Time: 15 minutes**

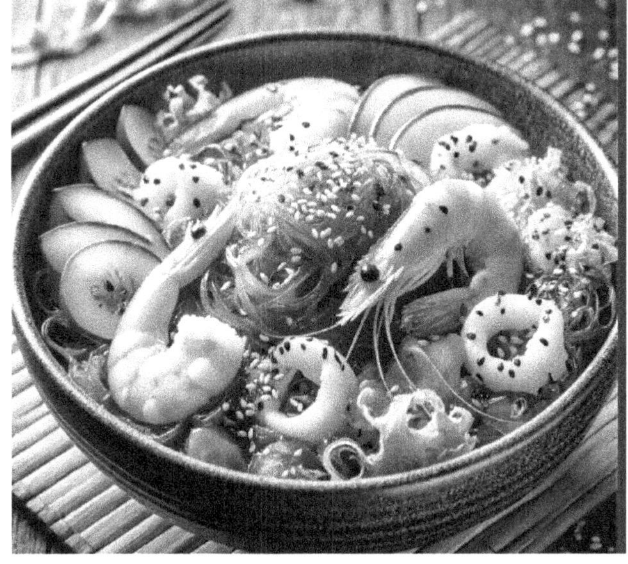

## 23. Italian Seafood Mix Fry

**Ingredients:**

- 1/2 lb shrimp, peeled and deveined
- 1/2 lb calamari, cleaned and sliced into rings
- 1/2 lb scallops
- 1/4 cup extra virgin olive oil
- 1/4 cup almond flour
- 1 teaspoon garlic powder
- 1 teaspoon dried oregano
- 1/2 teaspoon sea salt
- 1/4 teaspoon ground black pepper
- 1 lemon, cut into wedges

**Instructions:**

1. In a large bowl, mix the almond flour, garlic powder, dried oregano, sea salt, and black pepper.
2. Toss the shrimp, calamari, and scallops in the flour mixture to coat evenly.
3. In a large skillet, heat the olive oil over medium-high heat.
4. Add the seafood in batches, frying for 2-3 minutes on each side until golden and crispy.
5. Remove from the skillet and drain on paper towels.
6. Serve hot with lemon wedges.

**Nutrition Info (Per Serving):**

- Calories: 260
- Protein: 25g
- Carbohydrates: 4g
- Fat: 16g
- Fiber: 2g

**Serves: 4**
**Cooking Time: 20 minutes**

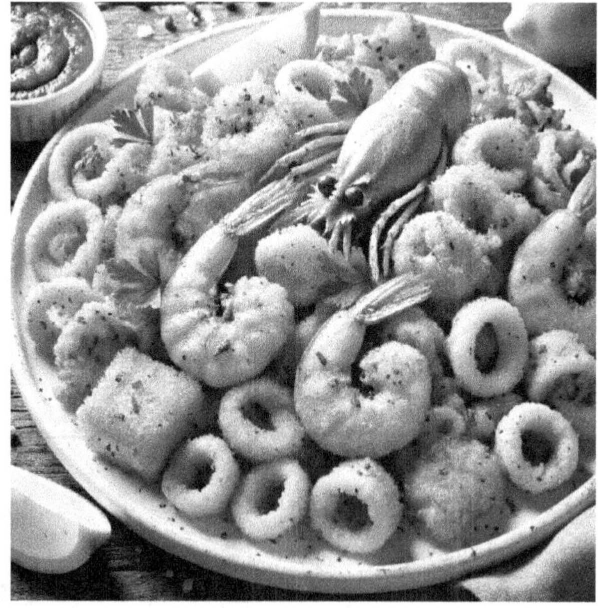

## 24. Poached Salmon with Dill Sauce

**Ingredients:**

- 4 salmon fillets (about 6 ounces each)
- 4 cups water
- 1/2 cup white wine
- 1 tablespoon sea salt
- 1 lemon, sliced
- 1 bunch fresh dill

Dill Sauce:

- 1/2 cup coconut yogurt
- 1 tablespoon fresh dill, chopped
- 1 tablespoon lemon juice
- 1 teaspoon Dijon mustard
- 1/4 teaspoon sea salt
- 1/4 teaspoon ground black pepper

**Instructions:**

1. In a large pot, combine the water, white wine, sea salt, lemon slices, and dill. Bring to a simmer.
2. Add the salmon fillets, ensuring they are fully submerged. Poach for 10-12 minutes, until the salmon is opaque and flakes easily.
3. Meanwhile, in a small bowl, mix the coconut yogurt, dill, lemon juice, Dijon mustard, sea salt, and black pepper to make the sauce.
4. Remove the salmon from the poaching liquid and serve hot with the dill sauce.

**Nutrition Info (Per Serving):**

- Calories: 280
- Protein: 34g
- Carbohydrates: 2g
- Fat: 14g
- Fiber: 0g

**Serves: 4**
**Cooking Time: 15 minutes**

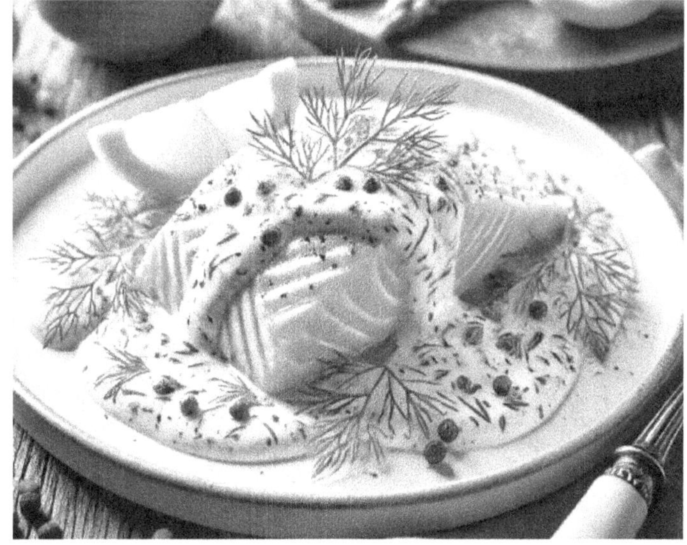

## 25. Lemon Garlic Poached Halibut

**Ingredients:**

- 4 halibut fillets (about 6 ounces each)
- 4 cups water
- 1/2 cup white wine
- 1 lemon, sliced
- 4 cloves garlic, sliced
- 1 tablespoon sea salt
- 1/4 cup fresh parsley, chopped

**Instructions:**

1. In a large pot, combine the water, white wine, lemon slices, garlic, and sea salt. Bring to a simmer.
2. Add the halibut fillets, ensuring they are fully submerged. Poach for 10-12 minutes, until the halibut is opaque and flakes easily.
3. Remove the halibut from the poaching liquid and serve hot, garnished with fresh parsley and additional lemon slices if desired.

**Nutrition Info (Per Serving):**

- Calories: 240
- Protein: 34g
- Carbohydrates: 2g
- Fat: 10g
- Fiber: 0g

**Serves: 4**
**Cooking Time: 15 minutes**

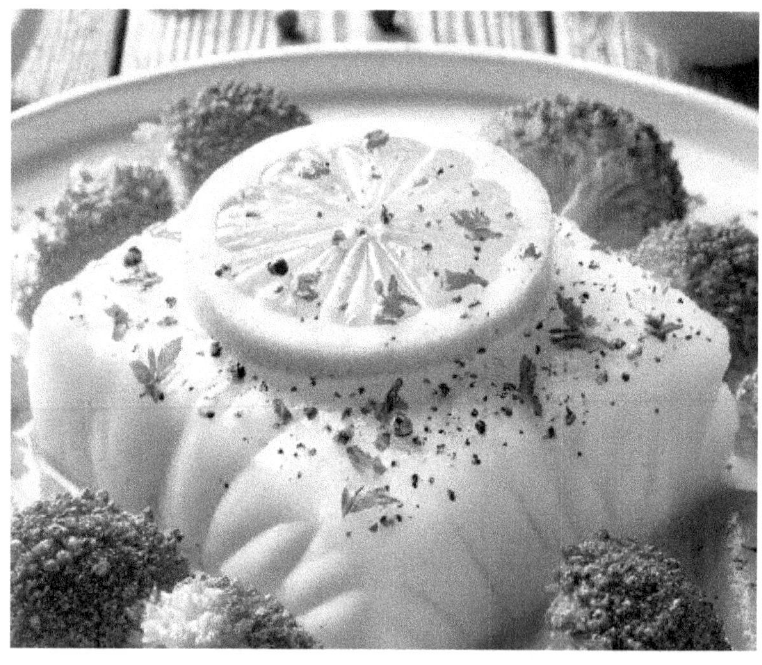

# *Poultry Recipes*

## 1. Herb-Roasted Chicken Thighs

**Ingredients:**

- 4 bone-in, skin-on chicken thighs
- 2 tablespoons extra virgin olive oil
- 1 tablespoon fresh rosemary, chopped
- 1 tablespoon fresh thyme, chopped
- 1 tablespoon fresh oregano, chopped
- 1 teaspoon sea salt
- 1/2 teaspoon ground black pepper
- 2 cloves garlic, minced
- Juice of 1 lemon

**Instructions:**

1. Preheat the oven to 400°F (200°C).
2. In a small bowl, combine the olive oil, rosemary, thyme, oregano, sea salt, black pepper, garlic, and lemon juice.
3. Rub the mixture evenly over the chicken thighs.
4. Place the chicken thighs on a baking sheet lined with parchment paper.
5. Roast in the preheated oven for 35-40 minutes, or until the chicken reaches an internal temperature of 165°F (74°C) and the skin is crispy.
6. Remove from the oven and let rest for 5 minutes before serving.

**Nutrition Info (Per Serving):**

- Calories: 280
- Protein: 25g
- Carbohydrates: 1g
- Fat: 20g
- Fiber: 0g

**Serves: 4**
**Cooking Time: 45 minutes**

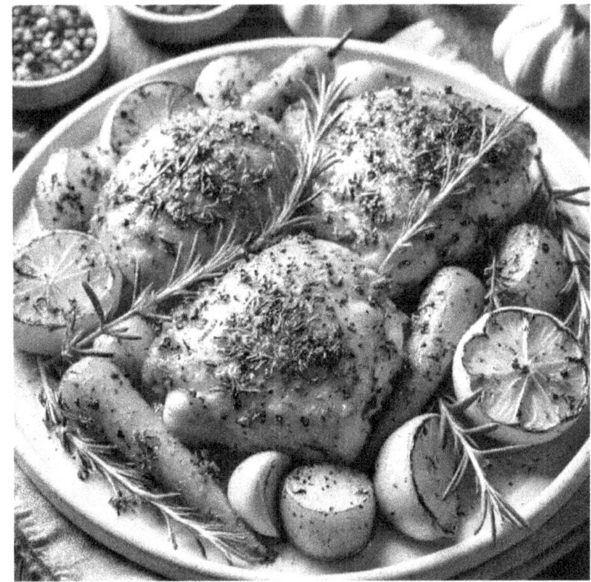

## 2. Lemon and Herb Turkey Breast

**Ingredients:**

- 1 boneless turkey breast (about 2 pounds)
- 3 tablespoons extra virgin olive oil
- 2 tablespoons fresh lemon juice
- 1 tablespoon fresh thyme, chopped
- 1 tablespoon fresh rosemary, chopped
- 2 cloves garlic, minced
- 1 teaspoon sea salt
- 1/2 teaspoon ground black pepper

**Instructions:**

1. Preheat the oven to 375°F (190°C).
2. In a small bowl, mix the olive oil, lemon juice, thyme, rosemary, garlic, sea salt, and black pepper.
3. Rub the mixture evenly over the turkey breast.
4. Place the turkey breast in a roasting pan.
5. Roast in the preheated oven for 45-55 minutes, or until the turkey reaches an internal temperature of 165°F (74°C).
6. Remove from the oven and let rest for 10 minutes before slicing and serving.

**Nutrition Info (Per Serving):**

- Calories: 240
- Protein: 32g
- Carbohydrates: 2g
- Fat: 10g
- Fiber: 0g

**Serves: 4**
**Cooking Time: 1 hour**

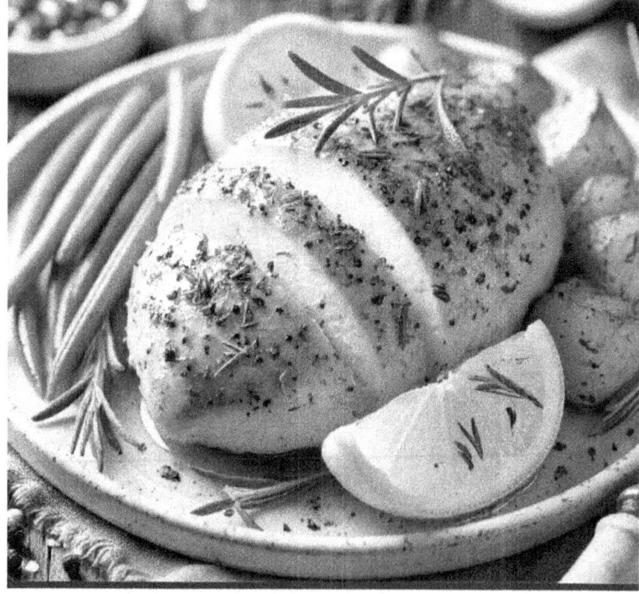

## 3. Garlic Butter Turkey Tenderloin

**Ingredients:**

- 1 lb turkey tenderloin
- 3 tablespoons unsalted butter, melted
- 2 cloves garlic, minced
- 1 tablespoon fresh parsley, chopped
- 1 teaspoon fresh thyme, chopped
- 1 teaspoon sea salt
- 1/2 teaspoon ground black pepper

**Instructions:**

1. Preheat the oven to 375°F (190°C).
2. In a small bowl, combine the melted butter, garlic, parsley, thyme, sea salt, and black pepper.
3. Rub the mixture evenly over the turkey tenderloin.
4. Place the turkey tenderloin in a baking dish.
5. Roast in the preheated oven for 25-30 minutes, or until the turkey reaches an internal temperature of 165°F (74°C).
6. Remove from the oven and let rest for 5 minutes before slicing and serving.

**Nutrition Info (Per Serving):**

- Calories: 220
- Protein: 26g
- Carbohydrates: 1g
- Fat: 12g
- Fiber: 0g

**Serves: 4**

**Cooking Time: 35 minutes**

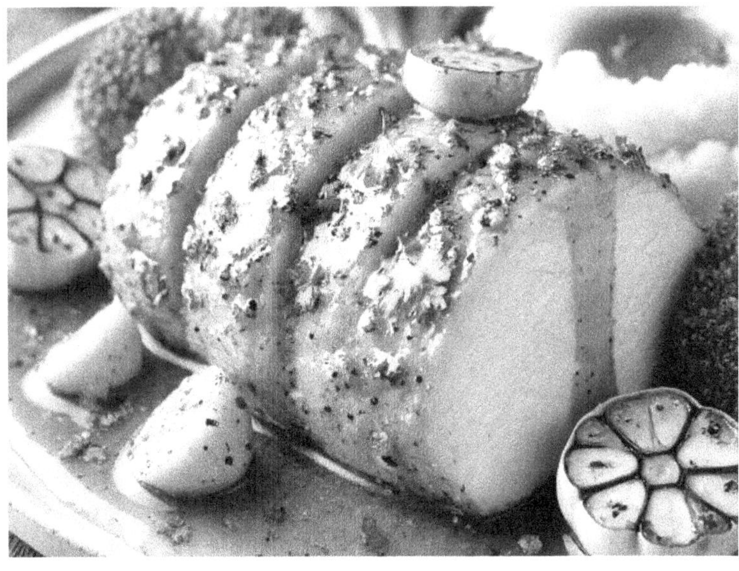

**4. Roast Chicken with Fennel and Carrots**

**Ingredients:**

- 1 whole chicken (about 4 pounds)
- 3 tablespoons extra virgin olive oil
- 1 tablespoon fresh rosemary, chopped
- 1 tablespoon fresh thyme, chopped
- 2 cloves garlic, minced
- 1 teaspoon sea salt
- 1/2 teaspoon ground black pepper
- 1 fennel bulb, sliced
- 4 carrots, peeled and sliced
- Juice of 1 lemon

**Instructions:**

1. Preheat the oven to 375°F (190°C).
2. In a small bowl, combine the olive oil, rosemary, thyme, garlic, sea salt, black pepper, and lemon juice.
3. Rub the mixture evenly over the chicken.
4. Place the chicken in a roasting pan and surround it with the fennel and carrots.
5. Roast in the preheated oven for 1 hour 15 minutes to 1 hour 30 minutes, or until the chicken reaches an internal temperature of 165°F (74°C).
6. Remove from the oven and let rest for 10 minutes before carving and serving.

**Nutrition Info (Per Serving):**

- Calories: 400
- Protein: 35g
- Carbohydrates: 10g
- Fat: 25g
- Fiber: 3g

**Serves: 6**

**Cooking Time: 1 hour 30 minutes**

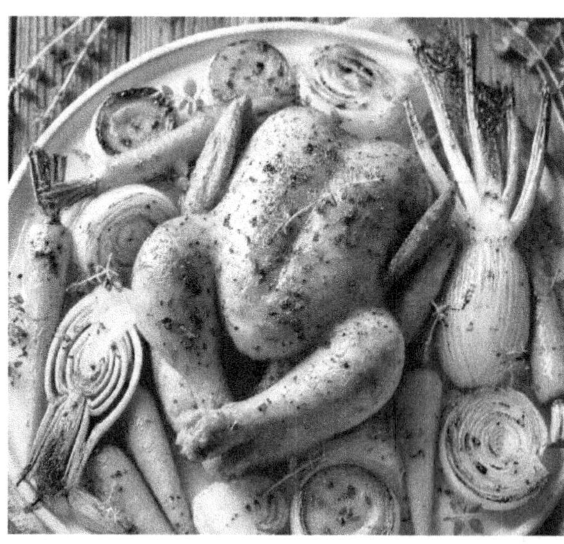

## 5. Grilled Chicken Kabobs

**Ingredients:**

- 1 lb boneless, skinless chicken breasts, cut into cubes
- 2 tablespoons extra virgin olive oil
- 1 tablespoon fresh lemon juice
- 2 cloves garlic, minced
- 1 tablespoon fresh oregano, chopped
- 1 teaspoon sea salt
- 1/2 teaspoon ground black pepper
- 1 red onion, cut into chunks
- 1 zucchini, cut into chunks

**Instructions:**

1. In a large bowl, mix the olive oil, lemon juice, garlic, oregano, sea salt, and black pepper.
2. Add the chicken cubes to the bowl, tossing to coat. Marinate for at least 30 minutes.
3. Preheat the grill to medium-high heat.
4. Thread the chicken, red onion, and zucchini onto skewers.
5. Grill the kabobs for 5-7 minutes on each side, until the chicken is cooked through and the vegetables are tender.
6. Serve hot.

**Nutrition Info (Per Serving):**

- Calories: 180
- Protein: 25g
- Carbohydrates: 6g
- Fat: 7g
- Fiber: 1g

**Serves: 4**

**Cooking Time: 15 minutes (plus marinating time)**

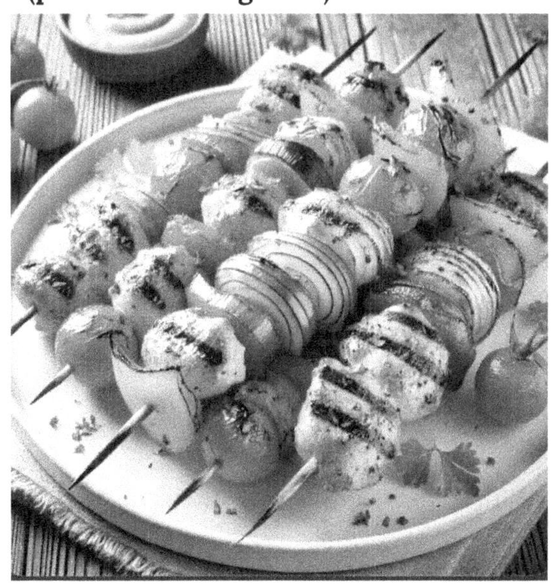

## 6. Barbecue Turkey Legs

**Ingredients:**

- 4 turkey legs
- 1/4 cup extra virgin olive oil
- 1/4 cup apple cider vinegar
- 2 cloves garlic, minced
- 1 tablespoon smoked paprika
- 1 tablespoon Dijon mustard
- 1 teaspoon sea salt
- 1/2 teaspoon ground black pepper

**Instructions:**

1. Preheat the grill to medium heat.
2. In a small bowl, mix the olive oil, apple cider vinegar, garlic, smoked paprika, Dijon mustard, sea salt, and black pepper.
3. Brush the mixture evenly over the turkey legs.
4. Grill the turkey legs for 30-40 minutes, turning occasionally, until the internal temperature reaches 165°F (74°C).
5. Serve hot.

**Nutrition Info (Per Serving):**

- Calories: 350
- Protein: 30g
- Carbohydrates: 2g
- Fat: 25g
- Fiber: 0g

**Serves: 4**

**Cooking Time: 40 minutes**

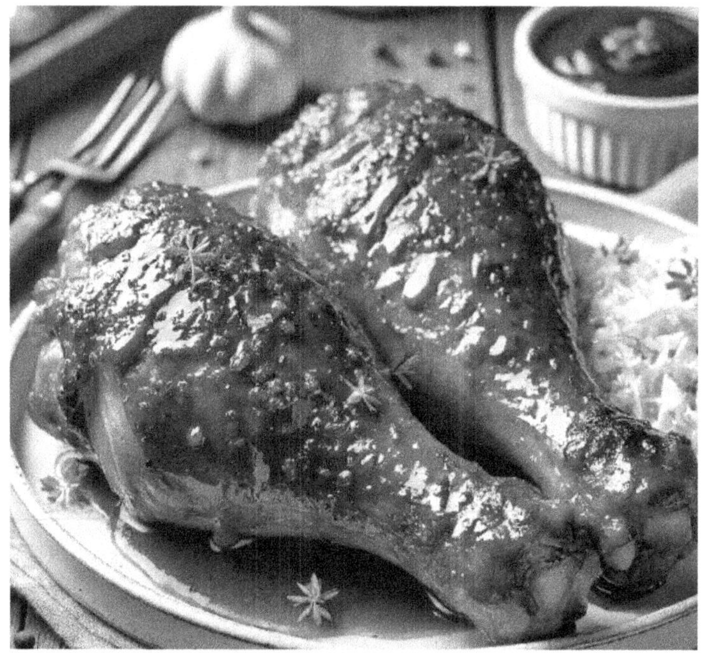

# 7. Lemon Pepper Chicken Wings

**Ingredients:**

- 2 lbs chicken wings
- 3 tablespoons extra virgin olive oil
- 2 tablespoons fresh lemon juice
- 1 tablespoon lemon zest
- 1 tablespoon freshly ground black pepper
- 1 teaspoon sea salt
- 1/4 teaspoon garlic powder

**Instructions:**

1. Preheat the oven to 400°F (200°C).
2. In a large bowl, combine the olive oil, lemon juice, lemon zest, black pepper, sea salt, and garlic powder.
3. Add the chicken wings to the bowl, tossing to coat.
4. Arrange the wings on a baking sheet lined with parchment paper.
5. Bake for 35-40 minutes, until the wings are crispy and cooked through.
6. Serve hot.

**Nutrition Info (Per Serving):**

- Calories: 300
- Protein: 25g
- Carbohydrates: 1g
- Fat: 22g
- Fiber: 0g

**Serves: 4**
**Cooking Time: 40 minutes**

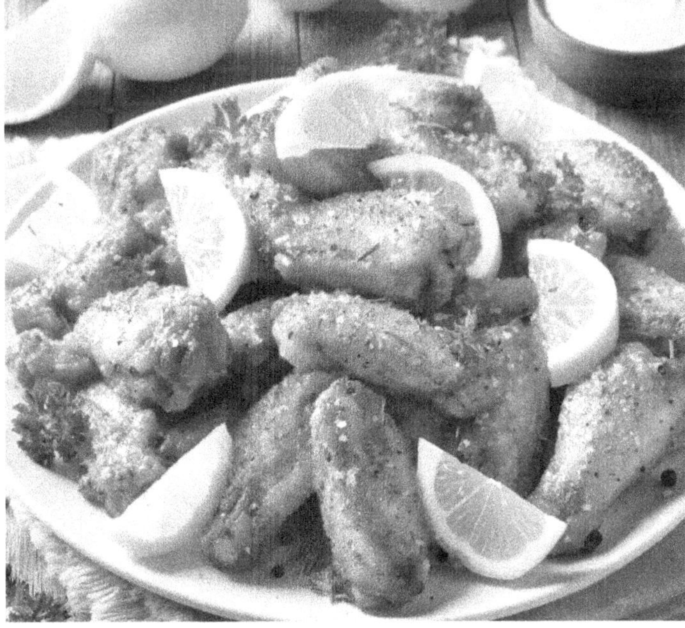

## 8. Smoked Turkey Breast

**Ingredients:**

- 1 boneless turkey breast (about 2 pounds)
- 2 tablespoons extra virgin olive oil
- 2 tablespoons apple cider vinegar
- 2 cloves garlic, minced
- 1 tablespoon smoked paprika
- 1 tablespoon fresh thyme, chopped
- 1 teaspoon sea salt
- 1/2 teaspoon ground black pepper

**Instructions:**

1. Preheat the smoker to 225°F (110°C).
2. In a small bowl, mix the olive oil, apple cider vinegar, garlic, smoked paprika, thyme, sea salt, and black pepper.
3. Rub the mixture evenly over the turkey breast.
4. Place the turkey breast in the smoker and smoke for 2-3 hours, until the internal temperature reaches 165°F (74°C).
5. Remove from the smoker and let rest for 10 minutes before slicing and serving.

**Nutrition Info (Per Serving):**

- Calories: 220
- Protein: 28g
- Carbohydrates: 1g
- Fat: 11g
- Fiber: 0g

**Serves: 4**
**Cooking Time: 3 hours**

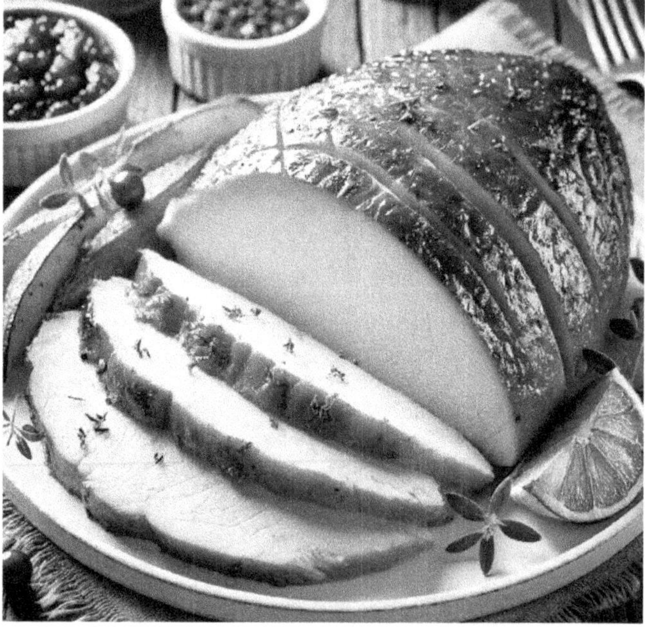

## 9. Chicken Piccata (No Flour)

**Ingredients:**

- 4 boneless, skinless chicken breasts
- 3 tablespoons extra virgin olive oil
- 1/4 cup fresh lemon juice
- 1/4 cup chicken broth
- 2 tablespoons capers, drained
- 2 cloves garlic, minced
- 1 tablespoon fresh parsley, chopped
- 1 teaspoon sea salt
- 1/2 teaspoon ground black pepper

**Instructions:**

1. In a large skillet, heat the olive oil over medium-high heat.
2. Season the chicken breasts with sea salt and black pepper.
3. Add the chicken to the skillet, cooking for 5-6 minutes on each side, until golden brown and cooked through. Remove from the skillet and set aside.
4. In the same skillet, add the garlic and sauté for 1 minute.
5. Add the lemon juice, chicken broth, and capers, simmering for 2-3 minutes until the sauce thickens slightly.
6. Return the chicken to the skillet, spooning the sauce over the top. Cook for another 2-3 minutes.
7. Garnish with fresh parsley and serve hot.

**Nutrition Info (Per Serving):**

- Calories: 250
- Protein: 28g
- Carbohydrates: 2g
- Fat: 14g
- Fiber: 0g

**Serves: 4**
**Cooking Time: 20 minutes**

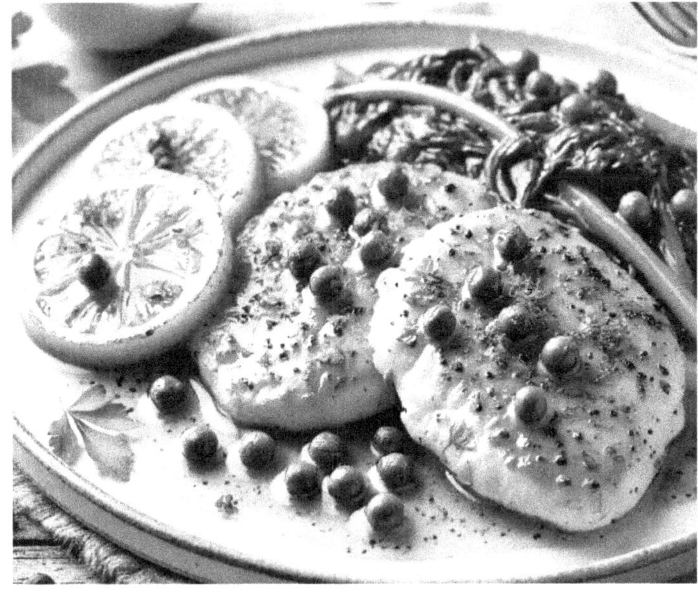

## 10. Turkey Scallopini

**Ingredients:**

- 1 lb turkey cutlets
- 3 tablespoons extra virgin olive oil
- 1/4 cup fresh lemon juice
- 1/4 cup chicken broth
- 2 cloves garlic, minced
- 1 tablespoon fresh parsley, chopped
- 1 teaspoon sea salt
- 1/2 teaspoon ground black pepper

**Instructions:**

1. In a large skillet, heat the olive oil over medium-high heat.
2. Season the turkey cutlets with sea salt and black pepper.
3. Add the turkey to the skillet, cooking for 3-4 minutes on each side, until golden brown and cooked through. Remove from the skillet and set aside.
4. In the same skillet, add the garlic and sauté for 1 minute.
5. Add the lemon juice and chicken broth, simmering for 2-3 minutes until the sauce thickens slightly.
6. Return the turkey to the skillet, spooning the sauce over the top. Cook for another 2-3 minutes.
7. Garnish with fresh parsley and serve hot.

**Nutrition Info (Per Serving):**

- Calories: 220
- Protein: 28g
- Carbohydrates: 2g
- Fat: 11g
- Fiber: 0g

**Serves: 4**
**Cooking Time: 15 minutes**

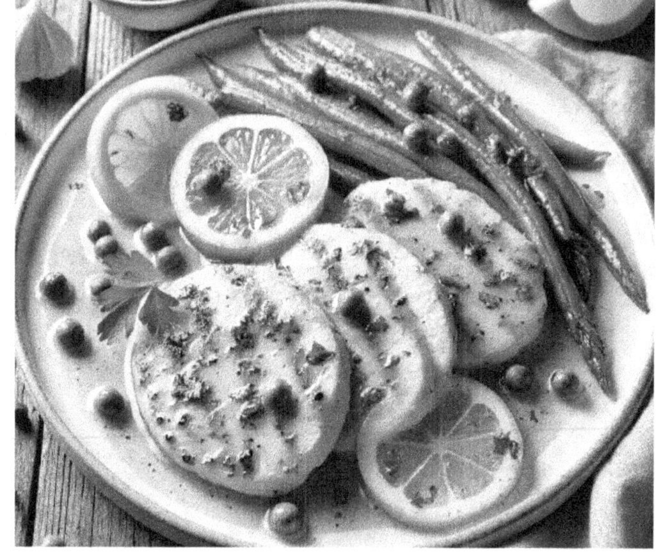

## 11. Sautéed Chicken Livers

**Ingredients:**

- 1 lb chicken livers, cleaned and trimmed
- 2 tablespoons extra virgin olive oil
- 1 large onion, finely chopped
- 2 cloves garlic, minced
- 1/4 cup fresh parsley, chopped
- 1 tablespoon fresh thyme, chopped
- 1 tablespoon fresh lemon juice
- 1 teaspoon sea salt
- 1/2 teaspoon ground black pepper

**Instructions:**

1. In a large skillet, heat the olive oil over medium heat.
2. Add the onion and garlic, sautéing until translucent, about 5 minutes.
3. Add the chicken livers, cooking for 5-7 minutes until browned and cooked through.
4. Stir in the parsley, thyme, lemon juice, sea salt, and black pepper. Cook for another 2 minutes.
5. Serve hot.

**Nutrition Info (Per Serving):**

- Calories: 180
- Protein: 24g
- Carbohydrates: 5g
- Fat: 7g
- Fiber: 1g

**Serves: 4**

**Cooking Time: 15 minutes**

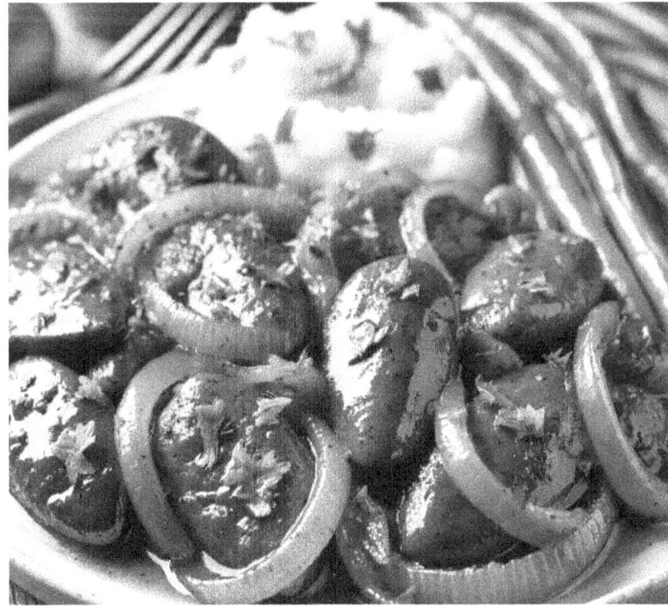

## 12. Chicken Saltimbocca

**Ingredients:**

- 4 boneless, skinless chicken breasts
- 8 slices prosciutto
- 8 fresh sage leaves
- 2 tablespoons extra virgin olive oil
- 1/4 cup chicken broth
- 1/4 cup dry white wine
- 2 cloves garlic, minced
- 1 tablespoon fresh lemon juice
- 1 teaspoon sea salt
- 1/2 teaspoon ground black pepper

**Instructions:**

1. Pound the chicken breasts to 1/4-inch thickness. Season with sea salt and black pepper.
2. Place 2 sage leaves on each chicken breast and wrap with 2 slices of prosciutto.
3. In a large skillet, heat the olive oil over medium-high heat. Add the chicken breasts and cook for 4-5 minutes on each side, until golden brown and cooked through.
4. Remove the chicken from the skillet and set aside.
5. In the same skillet, add the garlic and sauté for 1 minute.
6. Add the chicken broth and white wine, simmering for 2-3 minutes until the sauce thickens slightly.
7. Stir in the lemon juice and return the chicken to the skillet, spooning the sauce over the top. Cook for another 2 minutes.
8. Serve hot.

**Nutrition Info (Per Serving):**

- Calories: 260
- Protein: 34g
- Carbohydrates: 2g
- Fat: 12g
- Fiber: 0g

**Serves: 4**

**Cooking Time: 20 minutes**

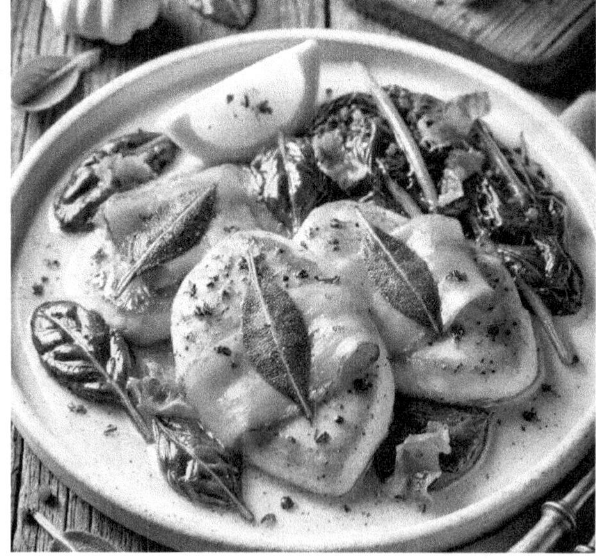

## 13. Chicken Vegetable Soup

**Ingredients:**

- 1 lb boneless, skinless chicken thighs, cut into chunks
- 2 tablespoons extra virgin olive oil
- 1 large onion, chopped
- 3 cloves garlic, minced
- 4 cups chicken broth
- 2 cups water
- 2 cups carrots, sliced
- 2 cups celery, sliced
- 1 cup green beans, chopped
- 1 teaspoon dried thyme
- 1 teaspoon sea salt
- 1/2 teaspoon ground black pepper
- 1/4 cup fresh parsley, chopped

**Instructions:**

1. In a large pot, heat the olive oil over medium heat. Add the onion and garlic, sautéing until translucent, about 5 minutes.
2. Add the chicken chunks and cook for another 5-7 minutes until browned.
3. Pour in the chicken broth and water, bringing to a boil.
4. Add the carrots, celery, green beans, thyme, sea salt, and black pepper. Reduce heat and simmer for 20-25 minutes until the vegetables are tender.
5. Stir in the fresh parsley.
6. Serve hot.

**Nutrition Info (Per Serving):**

- Calories: 220
- Protein: 25g
- Carbohydrates: 10g
- Fat: 10g
- Fiber: 3g

**Serves: 4**
**Cooking Time: 35 minutes**

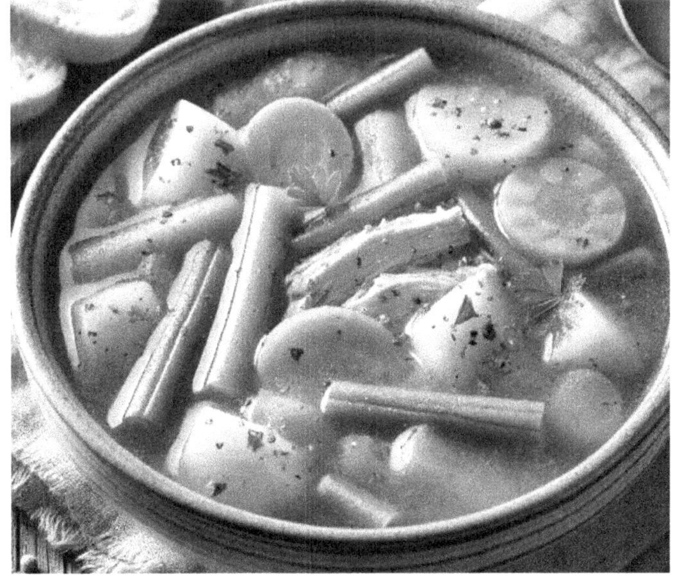

### 14. Chicken and Kale Stew

**Ingredients:**

- 1 lb boneless, skinless chicken thighs, cut into chunks
- 2 tablespoons extra virgin olive oil
- 1 large onion, chopped
- 3 cloves garlic, minced
- 4 cups chicken broth
- 2 cups water
- 4 cups kale, chopped
- 2 cups carrots, sliced
- 1 cup celery, sliced
- 1 teaspoon dried thyme
- 1 teaspoon sea salt
- 1/2 teaspoon ground black pepper
- 1/4 cup fresh parsley, chopped

**Instructions:**

1. In a large pot, heat the olive oil over medium heat. Add the onion and garlic, sautéing until translucent, about 5 minutes.
2. Add the chicken chunks and cook for another 5-7 minutes until browned.
3. Pour in the chicken broth and water, bringing to a boil.
4. Add the kale, carrots, celery, thyme, sea salt, and black pepper. Reduce heat and simmer for 25-30 minutes until the vegetables are tender.
5. Stir in the fresh parsley.
6. Serve hot.

**Nutrition Info (Per Serving):**

- Calories: 230
- Protein: 26g
- Carbohydrates: 12g
- Fat: 10g
- Fiber: 4g

**Serves: 4**

**Cooking Time: 40 minutes**

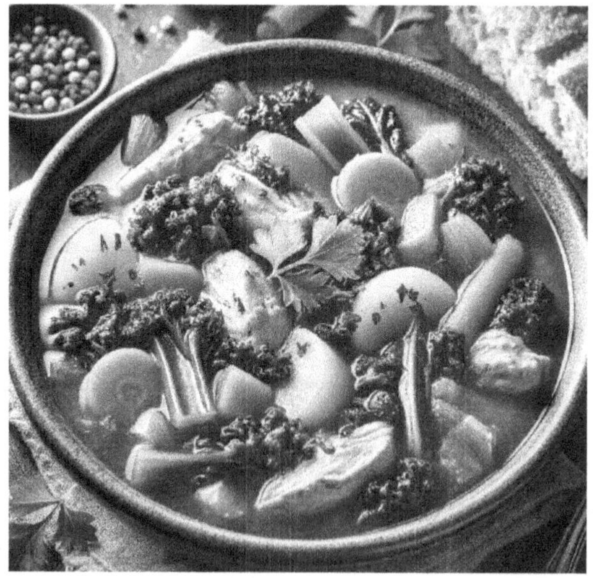

## 15. Herbed Turkey Soup with Root Vegetables

**Ingredients:**

- 1 lb turkey breast, cut into chunks
- 2 tablespoons extra virgin olive oil
- 1 large onion, chopped
- 3 cloves garlic, minced
- 4 cups turkey broth or chicken broth
- 2 cups water
- 2 cups carrots, sliced
- 2 cups parsnips, sliced
- 1 cup turnips, diced
- 1 teaspoon dried thyme
- 1 teaspoon dried rosemary
- 1 teaspoon sea salt
- 1/2 teaspoon ground black pepper
- 1/4 cup fresh parsley, chopped

**Instructions:**

1. In a large pot, heat the olive oil over medium heat. Add the onion and garlic, sautéing until translucent, about 5 minutes.
2. Add the turkey chunks and cook for another 5-7 minutes until browned.
3. Pour in the turkey broth and water, bringing to a boil.
4. Add the carrots, parsnips, turnips, thyme, rosemary, sea salt, and black pepper. Reduce heat and simmer for 25-30 minutes until the vegetables are tender.
5. Stir in the fresh parsley.
6. Serve hot.

**Nutrition Info (Per Serving):**

- Calories: 240
- Protein: 28g
- Carbohydrates: 14g
- Fat: 8g
- Fiber: 4g

**Serves: 4**
**Cooking Time: 40 minutes**

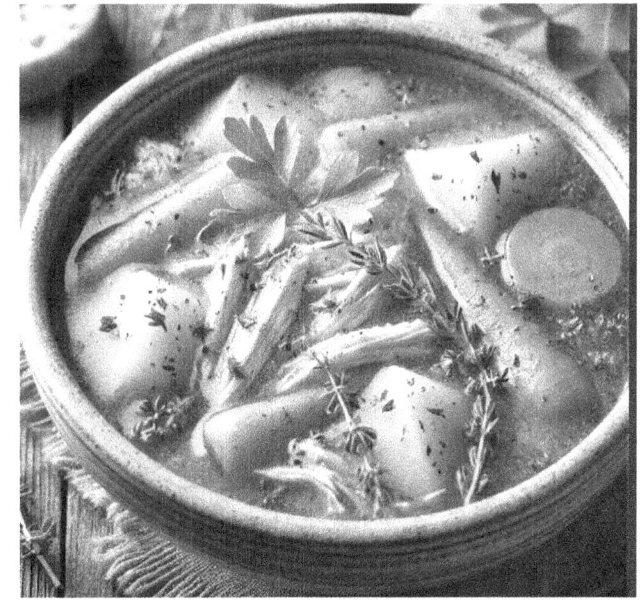

**16. Greek Lemon Chicken**

**Ingredients:**

- 4 boneless, skinless chicken breasts
- 1/4 cup extra virgin olive oil
- 1/4 cup fresh lemon juice
- 2 cloves garlic, minced
- 1 tablespoon dried oregano
- 1 teaspoon sea salt
- 1/2 teaspoon ground black pepper
- 1/4 cup fresh parsley, chopped

**Instructions:**

1. Preheat the oven to 375°F (190°C).
2. In a small bowl, mix the olive oil, lemon juice, garlic, oregano, sea salt, and black pepper.
3. Place the chicken breasts in a baking dish and pour the marinade over them.
4. Bake in the preheated oven for 25-30 minutes, or until the chicken reaches an internal temperature of 165°F (74°C).
5. Garnish with fresh parsley before serving.
6. Serve hot.

**Nutrition Info (Per Serving):**

- Calories: 250
- Protein: 28g
- Carbohydrates: 2g
- Fat: 14g
- Fiber: 0g

**Serves: 4**

**Cooking Time: 30 minutes**

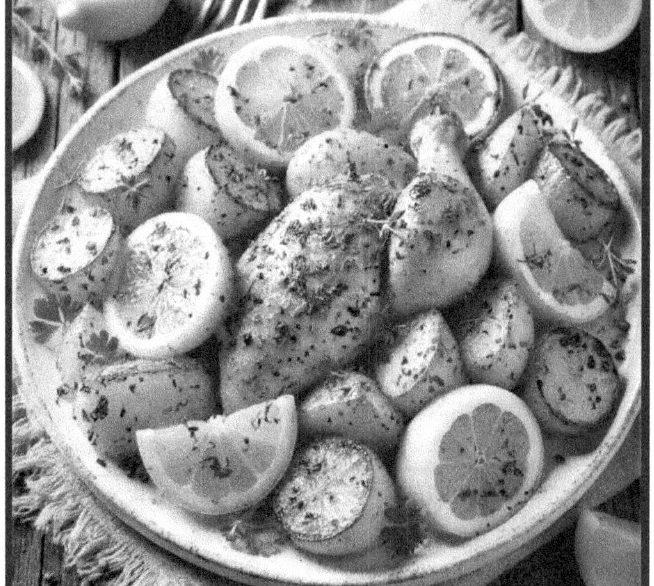

## 17. Thai Basil Turkey

**Ingredients:**

- 1 lb ground turkey
- 2 tablespoons extra virgin olive oil
- 1 large onion, chopped
- 2 cloves garlic, minced
- 1 tablespoon fresh ginger, grated
- 1 red bell pepper, chopped
- 1 cup fresh basil leaves, chopped
- 2 tablespoons coconut aminos
- 1 tablespoon fish sauce
- 1 teaspoon sea salt
- 1/2 teaspoon ground black pepper

**Instructions:**

1. In a large skillet, heat the olive oil over medium heat. Add the onion, garlic, and ginger, sautéing until the onion is translucent, about 5 minutes.
2. Add the ground turkey and cook until browned, breaking it up with a spoon, about 7-10 minutes.
3. Add the bell pepper and cook for another 3-4 minutes until tender.
4. Stir in the basil leaves, coconut aminos, fish sauce, sea salt, and black pepper. Cook for another 2 minutes.
5. Serve hot.

**Nutrition Info (Per Serving):**

- Calories: 220
- Protein: 25g
- Carbohydrates: 5g
- Fat: 12g
- Fiber: 1g

**Serves: 4**
**Cooking Time: 20 minutes**

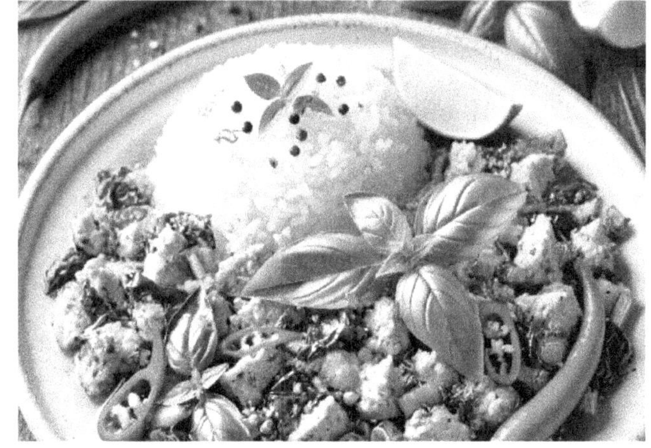

## 18. Turkey Cobb Salad

**Ingredients:**

- 1 lb cooked turkey breast, diced
- 6 cups mixed grccns (such as arugula, spinach, and kale)
- 1 avocado, sliced
- 1/2 cup red onion, thinly sliced
- 1/2 cup cucumber, sliced
- 1/4 cup fresh parsley, chopped
- 1/4 cup extra virgin olive oil
- 2 tablespoons apple cider vinegar
- 1 teaspoon Dijon mustard
- 1 teaspoon sea salt
- 1/2 teaspoon ground black pepper

**Instructions:**

1. In a large salad bowl, combine the mixed greens, turkey, avocado, red onion, cucumber, and parsley.
2. In a small bowl, whisk together the olive oil, apple cider vinegar, Dijon mustard, sea salt, and black pepper.
3. Drizzle the dressing over the salad and toss gently to combine.
4. Serve immediately.

**Nutrition Info (Per Serving):**

- Calories: 300
- Protein: 30g
- Carbohydrates: 10g
- Fat: 18g
- Fiber: 6g

**Serves: 4**
**Cooking Time: 10 minutes**

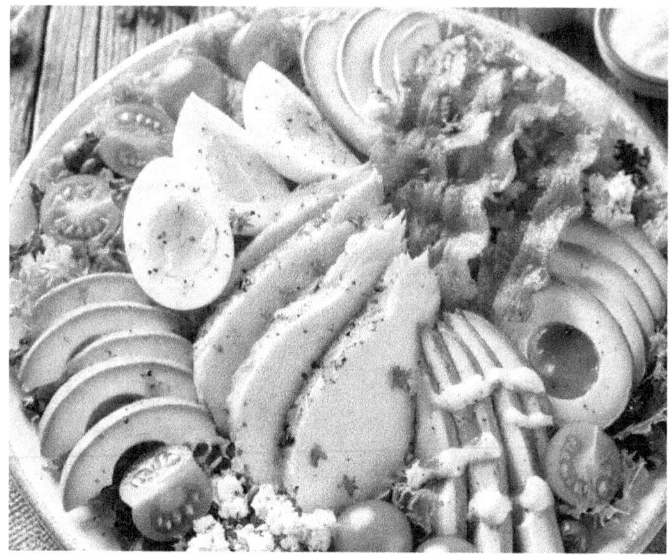

## 19. Chicken Meatballs with Herb Sauce

**Ingredients:**

- 1 lb ground chicken
- 1/4 cup almond flour
- 1 egg, beaten
- 2 cloves garlic, minced
- 1 tablespoon fresh parsley, chopped
- 1 tablespoon fresh thyme, chopped
- 1 teaspoon sea salt
- 1/2 teaspoon ground black pepper
- 2 tablespoons extra virgin olive oil

**Herb Sauce:**

- 1/4 cup extra virgin olive oil
- 2 tablespoons fresh lemon juice
- 1 tablespoon fresh basil, chopped
- 1 tablespoon fresh dill, chopped
- 1 teaspoon Dijon mustard
- 1 teaspoon sea salt
- 1/4 teaspoon ground black pepper

**Instructions:**

1. In a large bowl, combine the ground chicken, almond flour, egg, garlic, parsley, thyme, sea salt, and black pepper. Mix well.
2. Form the mixture into small meatballs.
3. In a large skillet, heat the olive oil over medium heat. Add the meatballs and cook for 6-8 minutes on each side, until browned and cooked through.
4. In a small bowl, whisk together the olive oil, lemon juice, basil, dill, Dijon mustard, sea salt, and black pepper to make the herb sauce.
5. Drizzle the herb sauce over the meatballs before serving.
6. Serve hot.

**Nutrition Info (Per Serving):**

- Calories: 280
- Protein: 24g
- Carbohydrates: 4g
- Fat: 18g
- Fiber: 2g

**Serves: 4**

**Cooking Time: 20 minutes**

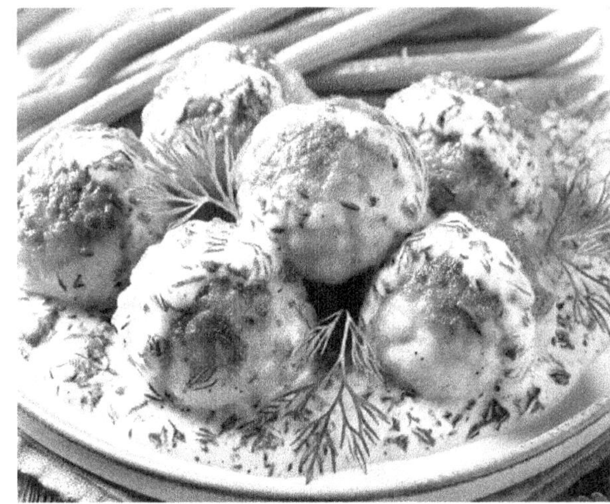

## 20. Buffalo Chicken Stuffed Celery (No Cheese)

**Ingredients:**

- 2 cups cooked chicken breast, shredded
- 1/4 cup buffalo saucc
- 1/4 cup coconut yogurt
- 1 tablespoon fresh chives, chopped
- 8 large celery stalks, cut into 3-inch pieces

**Instructions:**

1. In a medium bowl, combine the shredded chicken, buffalo sauce, coconut yogurt, and chives. Mix well.
2. Fill each celery piece with the buffalo chicken mixture.
3. Serve immediately.

**Nutrition Info (Per Serving):**

- Calories: 100
- Protein: 12g
- Carbohydrates: 4g
- Fat: 5g
- Fiber: 1g

**Serves: 4**

**Cooking Time: 10 minutes**

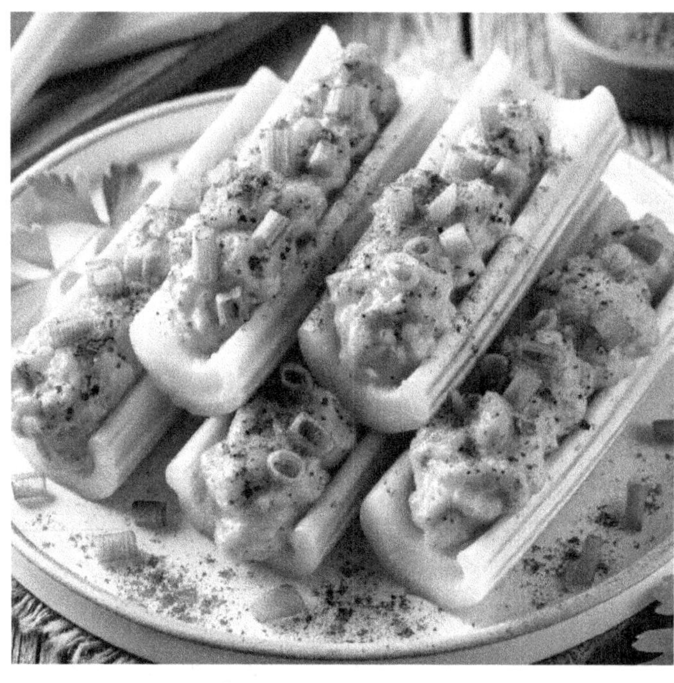

## 21. Pan-Seared Chicken with Rosemary

**Ingredients:**

- 4 boneless, skinless chicken breasts
- 3 tablespoons extra virgin olive oil
- 2 cloves garlic, minced
- 1 tablespoon fresh rosemary, chopped
- 1 teaspoon sea salt
- 1/2 teaspoon ground black pepper
- Juice of 1 lemon

**Instructions:**

1. In a small bowl, mix the olive oil, garlic, rosemary, sea salt, black pepper, and lemon juice.
2. Rub the mixture evenly over the chicken breasts.
3. In a large skillet, heat a little extra olive oil over medium-high heat.
4. Add the chicken breasts and cook for 5-6 minutes on each side, until golden brown and cooked through.
5. Serve hot.

**Nutrition Info (Per Serving):**

- Calories: 240
- Protein: 28g
- Carbohydrates: 1g
- Fat: 14g
- Fiber: 0g

**Serves: 4**
**Cooking Time: 15 minutes**

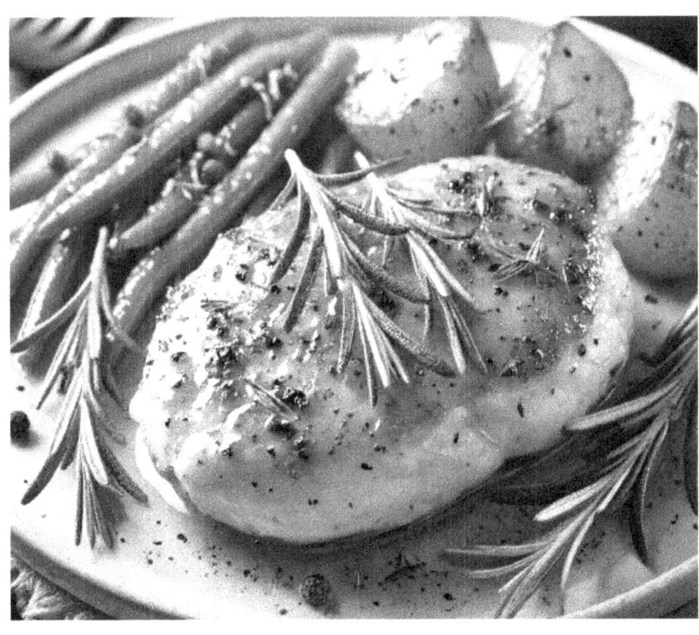

# 10-WEEK MEAL PLAN

## Week 1

Monday
- Breakfast: Almond Flour Pancakes
- Lunch: Greek Lemon Chicken with a side of steamed broccoli
- Dinner: Fisherman's Stew with Halibut

Tuesday
- Breakfast: Almond Butter Banana Smoothie
- Lunch: Turkey Cobb Salad
- Dinner: Chicken Vegetable Soup

Wednesday
- Breakfast: Flaxseed Porridge
- Lunch: Grilled Mahi-Mahi with Lime and sautéed spinach
- Dinner: Thai Basil Turkey

Thursday
- Breakfast: Baked Coconut Custard
- Lunch: Lemon and Herb Turkey Breast with a side of roasted asparagus
- Dinner: Chicken and Kale Stew

Friday
- Breakfast: Pistachio and Pumpkin Seed Granola
- Lunch: Shrimp Salad with Mixed Greens
- Dinner: Indian Fish Curry with Coconut Milk

Saturday
- Breakfast: Radish and Smoked Salmon Plate
- Lunch: Chicken Meatballs with Herb Sauce and steamed green beans
- Dinner: Oven-Roasted Trout with Thyme

Sunday
- Breakfast: Sautéed Chicken Livers
- Lunch: Grilled Chicken Kabobs with a side of cucumber salad
- Dinner: Herb-Roasted Chicken Thighs with roasted carrots

## Week 2

Monday
- Breakfast: Kale Caesar Salad
- Lunch: Poached Salmon with Dill Sauce and steamed cauliflower
- Dinner: Buffalo Chicken Stuffed Celery

Tuesday
- Breakfast: Sautéed Kale with Poached Eggs
- Lunch: Greek Style Grilled Octopus with a side of roasted zucchini
- Dinner: Chicken Piccata (No Flour) with a side of mashed turnips

Wednesday
- Breakfast: Lemon and Herb Chicken Drumsticks
- Lunch: Crab Salad with Celery
- Dinner: Barbecue Turkey Legs with steamed broccoli

Thursday
- Breakfast: Coconut Almond Bars
- Lunch: Japanese Seaweed and Seafood Salad
- Dinner: Smoked Turkey Breast with a side of roasted Brussels sprouts

Friday
- Breakfast: Olive Tapenade with Endive Leaves
- Lunch: Char-Grilled Octopus with Olive Oil
- Dinner: Turkey Scallopini with a side of sautéed spinach

Saturday
- Breakfast: Radish Raita
- Lunch: Shrimp Broth with Fennel
- Dinner: Grilled Tuna Steaks with Olive Oil and a side of steamed asparagus

Sunday
- Breakfast: Celery Root Remoulade
- Lunch: Chicken Saltimbocca with a side of roasted vegetables
- Dinner: Roasted Garlic Spread with grilled chicken breasts

## Week 3

Monday
- Breakfast: Herbal Tea with Coconut Oil
- Lunch: Sardines Fried in Olive Oil with a side of arugula salad
- Dinner: Herbed Turkey Soup with Root Vegetables

Tuesday
- Breakfast: Pumpkin Seed Muesli
- Lunch: Turkey Scallopini with a side of sautéed green beans
- Dinner: Barbecue Shrimp Skewers with a side of grilled zucchini

Wednesday
- Breakfast: Sautéed Kale with Poached Eggs
- Lunch: Beef and Vegetable Breakfast Soup
- Dinner: Pan-Seared Chicken with Rosemary and roasted carrots

Thursday
- Breakfast: Broccoli Almond Salad
- Lunch: Tuna Tartare with Avocado and a side of mixed greens
- Dinner: Chicken and Kale Stew

Friday

- Breakfast: Flaxseed Porridge
- Lunch: Grilled Salmon with Dill and a side of steamed broccoli
- Dinner: Fisherman's Stew with Halibut

Saturday

- Breakfast: Almond Flour Pancakes
- Lunch: Chicken Piccata (No Flour) with a side of roasted asparagus
- Dinner: Shrimp Broth with Fennel

Sunday

- Breakfast: Baked Coconut Custard
- Lunch: Char-Grilled Octopus with Olive Oil and a side of cucumber salad
- Dinner: Roast Chicken with Fennel and Carrots

## Week 4

Monday

- Breakfast: Watercress Soup
- Lunch: Greek Lemon Chicken with a side of steamed cauliflower
- Dinner: Shrimp Sautéed with Spinach

Tuesday

- Breakfast: Mustard Greens Spicy Stir Fry
- Lunch: Crab Stir-Fry with Ginger
- Dinner: Chicken Vegetable Soup

Wednesday

- Breakfast: Collard Greens with Garlic
- Lunch: Smoked Salmon Salad with Arugula
- Dinner: Buffalo Chicken Stuffed Celery

Thursday

- Breakfast: Swiss Chard and Pine Nuts
- Lunch: Indian Spiced Cauliflower (Gobi Masala)
- Dinner: Poached Salmon with Dill Sauce

Friday

- Breakfast: Tuna and Olive Salad
- Lunch: Grilled Chicken Kabobs with a side of roasted vegetables
- Dinner: Thai Basil Turkey

Saturday

- Breakfast: Mustard Greens and Bacon Stir-Fry
- Lunch: Shrimp Salad with Mixed Greens
- Dinner: Chicken Meatballs with Herb Sauce and steamed broccoli

Sunday
- Breakfast: Celery Root Remoulade
- Lunch: Italian Seafood Mix Fry with a side of arugula salad
- Dinner: Chicken and Kale Stew

## Week 5

Monday
- Breakfast: Radish and Smoked Salmon Plate
- Lunch: Grilled Tuna Steaks with Olive Oil and a side of sautéed spinach
- Dinner: Herbed Turkey Soup with Root Vegetables

Tuesday
- Breakfast: Carrot and Cucumber Nori Rolls
- Lunch: Fisherman's Stew with Halibut
- Dinner: Chicken Piccata (No Flour) with a side of roasted carrots

Wednesday
- Breakfast: Sautéed Kale with Poached Eggs
- Lunch: Beef and Vegetable Breakfast Soup
- Dinner: Grilled Mahi-Mahi with Lime and a side of steamed asparagus

Thursday
- Breakfast: Radish Raita
- Lunch: Char-Grilled Octopus with Olive Oil
- Dinner: Shrimp Broth with Fennel

Friday
- Breakfast: Almond Butter Banana Smoothie
- Lunch: Grilled Chicken Kabobs with a side of roasted zucchini
- Dinner: Poached Salmon with Dill Sauce

Saturday
- Breakfast: Pistachio and Pumpkin Seed Granola
- Lunch: Crab Salad with Celery
- Dinner: Greek Style Grilled Octopus with a side of cucumber salad

Sunday
- Breakfast: Collard Greens with Garlic
- Lunch: Shrimp Sautéed with Spinach
- Dinner: Roast Chicken with Fennel and Carrots

## Week 6

Monday
- Breakfast: Cinnamon Coconut Latte
- Lunch: Hard-Boiled Eggs with Olive Oil Drizzle and a side of arugula
- Dinner: Barbecue Turkey Legs with steamed Brussels sprouts

Tuesday
- Breakfast: Kale and Olive Oil Smoothie
- Lunch: Ceviche with Snapper and Lime
- Dinner: Lemon and Herb Turkey Breast with roasted fennel

Wednesday
- Breakfast: Swiss Chard and Pine Nuts
- Lunch: Broccoli Rabe with Olives
- Dinner: Pan-Seared Chicken with Rosemary and sautéed green beans

Thursday
- Breakfast: Flaxseed Porridge
- Lunch: Smoked Turkey Breast with a side of kale salad
- Dinner: Fisherman's Stew with Halibut

Friday
- Breakfast: Watercress Soup
- Lunch: Garlic and Herb Roasted Shallots with grilled chicken
- Dinner: Shrimp Broth with Fennel

Saturday
- Breakfast: Celery and Almond Butter
- Lunch: Crab Stir-Fry with Ginger
- Dinner: Poached Salmon with Dill Sauce

Sunday
- Breakfast: Baked Coconut Custard
- Lunch: Radish and Smoked Salmon Plate
- Dinner: Greek Lemon Chicken with a side of roasted carrots

## Week 7

Monday
- Breakfast: Olive Tapenade with Endive Leaves
- Lunch: Shrimp Salad with Mixed Greens
- Dinner: Chicken and Kale Stew

Tuesday
- Breakfast: Pistachio and Pumpkin Seed Granola
- Lunch: Italian Seafood Mix Fry with a side of cucumber salad
- Dinner: Grilled Tuna Steaks with Olive Oil

Wednesday
- Breakfast: Broccoli Almond Salad
- Lunch: Grilled Mahi-Mahi with Lime
- Dinner: Chicken Piccata (No Flour) with steamed broccoli

Thursday

- Breakfast: Hard-Boiled Eggs with Olive Oil Drizzle
- Lunch: Char-Grilled Octopus with Olive Oil
- Dinner: Buffalo Chicken Stuffed Celery

Friday

- Breakfast: Sautéed Kale with Poached Eggs
- Lunch: Sardines Fried in Olive Oil with a side of mixed greens
- Dinner: Chicken Meatballs with Herb Sauce and steamed green beans

Saturday

- Breakfast: Swiss Chard and Pine Nuts
- Lunch: Ceviche with Snapper and Lime
- Dinner: Indian Fish Curry with Coconut Milk

Sunday

- Breakfast: Radish and Smoked Salmon Plate
- Lunch: Shrimp Sautéed with Spinach
- Dinner: Herbed Turkey Soup with Root Vegetables

## Week 8

Monday

- Breakfast: Olive Tapenade with Endive Leaves
- Lunch: Lemon and Herb Turkey Breast with roasted fennel
- Dinner: Shrimp Broth with Fennel

Tuesday

- Breakfast: Kale and Olive Oil Smoothie
- Lunch: Poached Salmon with Dill Sauce and steamed broccoli
- Dinner: Chicken and Kale Stew

Wednesday

- Breakfast: Flaxseed Porridge
- Lunch: Barbecue Shrimp Skewers with a side of grilled zucchini
- Dinner: Pan-Seared Chicken with Rosemary

Thursday

- Breakfast: Pistachio and Pumpkin Seed Granola
- Lunch: Broccoli Rabe with Olives
- Dinner: Grilled Tuna Steaks with Olive Oil

Friday

- Breakfast: Watercress Soup
- Lunch: Crab Salad with Celery
- Dinner: Chicken Meatballs with Herb Sauce

Saturday

- Breakfast: Swiss Chard and Pine Nuts
- Lunch: Indian Spiced Cauliflower (Gobi Masala)
- Dinner: Fisherman's Stew with Halibut

Sunday

- Breakfast: Radish and Smoked Salmon Plate
- Lunch: Smoked Turkey Breast with a side of arugula salad
- Dinner: Greek Lemon Chicken

## Week 9

Monday

- Breakfast: Almond Flour Pancakes
- Lunch: Shrimp Salad with Mixed Greens
- Dinner: Chicken Piccata (No Flour)

Tuesday

- Breakfast: Sautéed Kale with Poached Eggs
- Lunch: Char-Grilled Octopus with Olive Oil
- Dinner: Poached Salmon with Dill Sauce

Wednesday

- Breakfast: Hard-Boiled Eggs with Olive Oil Drizzle
- Lunch: Grilled Mahi-Mahi with Lime
- Dinner: Chicken and Kale Stew

Thursday

- Breakfast: Flaxseed Porridge
- Lunch: Ceviche with Snapper and Lime
- Dinner: Pan-Seared Chicken with Rosemary

Friday

- Breakfast: Kale and Olive Oil Smoothie
- Lunch: Broccoli Rabe with Olives
- Dinner: Barbecue Turkey Legs

Saturday

- Breakfast: Olive Tapenade with Endive Leaves
- Lunch: Crab Stir-Fry with Ginger
- Dinner: Indian Fish Curry with Coconut Milk

Sunday

- Breakfast: Pistachio and Pumpkin Seed Granola
- Lunch: Smoked Salmon Salad with Arugula
- Dinner: Herbed Turkey Soup with Root Vegetables

# Week 10

Monday
- Breakfast: Swiss Chard and Pine Nuts
- Lunch: Grilled Tuna Steaks with Olive Oil
- Dinner: Chicken Meatballs with Herb Sauce

Tuesday
- Breakfast: Radish and Smoked Salmon Plate
- Lunch: Shrimp Broth with Fennel
- Dinner: Chicken and Kale Stew

Wednesday
- Breakfast: Watercress Soup
- Lunch: Char-Grilled Octopus with Olive Oil
- Dinner: Pan-Seared Chicken with Rosemary

Thursday
- Breakfast: Sautéed Kale with Poached Eggs
- Lunch: Crab Salad with Celery
- Dinner: Poached Salmon with Dill Sauce

Friday
- Breakfast: Flaxseed Porridge
- Lunch: Sardines Fried in Olive Oil with a side of mixed greens
- Dinner: Indian Fish Curry with Coconut Milk

Saturday
- Breakfast: Hard-Boiled Eggs with Olive Oil Drizzle
- Lunch: Barbecue Shrimp Skewers with a side of grilled zucchini
- Dinner: Fisherman's Stew with Halibut

Sunday
- Breakfast: Pistachio and Pumpkin Seed Granola
- Lunch: Greek Lemon Chicken with roasted carrots
- Dinner: Herbed Turkey Soup with Root Vegetables

# WEEKLY MEAL PLANNER  +  WORKBOOK

|  | BREAKFAST | LUNCH | DINNER | SNACKS |
|---|---|---|---|---|
| MONDAY |  |  |  |  |
| TUESDAY |  |  |  |  |
| WEDNESDAY |  |  |  |  |
| THURSDAY |  |  |  |  |
| FRIDAY |  |  |  |  |
| SATURDAY |  |  |  |  |
| SUNDAY |  |  |  |  |

**Why have you decided to start a lectin-free diet?**
**Reflect on your motivations and goals for adopting this dietary change.**

# WEEKLY MEAL PLANNER + WORKBOOK

|  | BREAKFAST | LUNCH | DINNER | SNACKS |
|---|---|---|---|---|
| MONDAY |  |  |  |  |
| TUESDAY |  |  |  |  |
| WEDNESDAY |  |  |  |  |
| THURSDAY |  |  |  |  |
| FRIDAY |  |  |  |  |
| SATURDAY |  |  |  |  |
| SUNDAY |  |  |  |  |

How do you currently feel about your health and energy levels? Describe your physical and mental state before starting the diet.

# *WEEKLY MEAL PLANNER + WORKBOOK*

| | BREAKFAST | LUNCH | DINNER | SNACKS |
|---|---|---|---|---|
| MONDAY | | | | |
| TUESDAY | | | | |
| WEDNESDAY | | | | |
| THURSDAY | | | | |
| FRIDAY | | | | |
| SATURDAY | | | | |
| SUNDAY | | | | |

**What are some of your favorite meals or snacks that you hope to find lectin-free alternatives for?**

- **List your top three meals or snacks and think about how they can be adapted.**

# *WEEKLY MEAL PLANNER + WORKBOOK*

|  | BREAKFAST | LUNCH | DINNER | SNACKS |
|---|---|---|---|---|
| MONDAY |  |  |  |  |
| TUESDAY |  |  |  |  |
| WEDNESDAY |  |  |  |  |
| THURSDAY |  |  |  |  |
| FRIDAY |  |  |  |  |
| SATURDAY |  |  |  |  |
| SUNDAY |  |  |  |  |

Have you identified any high-lectin foods in your current diet? Make a list of foods you commonly eat that are high in lectins.

# WEEKLY MEAL PLANNER  +  WORKBOOK

|  | BREAKFAST | LUNCH | DINNER | SNACKS |
|---|---|---|---|---|
| MONDAY |  |  |  |  |
| TUESDAY |  |  |  |  |
| WEDNESDAY |  |  |  |  |
| THURSDAY |  |  |  |  |
| FRIDAY |  |  |  |  |
| SATURDAY |  |  |  |  |
| SUNDAY |  |  |  |  |

**What are your main concerns about starting a lectin-free diet? Write down any worries or questions you have.**

# WEEKLY MEAL PLANNER + WORKBOOK

| | BREAKFAST | LUNCH | DINNER | SNACKS |
|---|---|---|---|---|
| MONDAY | | | | |
| TUESDAY | | | | |
| WEDNESDAY | | | | |
| THURSDAY | | | | |
| FRIDAY | | | | |
| SATURDAY | | | | |
| SUNDAY | | | | |

What steps will you take to make grocery shopping easier on a lectin-free diet? Think about how you will approach shopping for lectin-free foods.

# WEEKLY MEAL PLANNER + WORKBOOK

| | BREAKFAST | LUNCH | DINNER | SNACKS |
|---|---|---|---|---|
| MONDAY | | | | |
| TUESDAY | | | | |
| WEDNESDAY | | | | |
| THURSDAY | | | | |
| FRIDAY | | | | |
| SATURDAY | | | | |
| SUNDAY | | | | |

**What support systems do you have in place to help you succeed? Identify friends, family, or online communities that can provide support and encouragement.**

........................................................................................................................

........................................................................................................................

........................................................................................................................

........................................................................................................................

........................................................................................................................

# WEEKLY MEAL PLANNER  +  WORKBOOK

|  | BREAKFAST | LUNCH | DINNER | SNACKS |
|---|---|---|---|---|
| MONDAY |  |  |  |  |
| TUESDAY |  |  |  |  |
| WEDNESDAY |  |  |  |  |
| THURSDAY |  |  |  |  |
| FRIDAY |  |  |  |  |
| SATURDAY |  |  |  |  |
| SUNDAY |  |  |  |  |

How will you measure the success of your lectin-free diet? Define what success looks like for you and how you will track your progress.

# WEEKLY MEAL PLANNER + WORKBOOK

|  | BREAKFAST | LUNCH | DINNER | SNACKS |
|---|---|---|---|---|
| MONDAY | | | | |
| TUESDAY | | | | |
| WEDNESDAY | | | | |
| THURSDAY | | | | |
| FRIDAY | | | | |
| SATURDAY | | | | |
| SUNDAY | | | | |

**What are some lectin-free recipes you are excited to try? List a few recipes that appeal to you and why you chose them.**

# WEEKLY MEAL PLANNER + WORKBOOK

|  | BREAKFAST | LUNCH | DINNER | SNACKS |
|---|---|---|---|---|
| MONDAY | | | | |
| TUESDAY | | | | |
| WEDNESDAY | | | | |
| THURSDAY | | | | |
| FRIDAY | | | | |
| SATURDAY | | | | |
| SUNDAY | | | | |

What kitchen tools or equipment might help you prepare lectin-free meals more efficiently?
Consider any gadgets or tools that could make cooking easier and more enjoyable.

# Scan the QR code below to get a surprise bonus!